Dr. med. Uwe Auf der Strasse

Shadow Disease

chronic active Toxoplasmosis

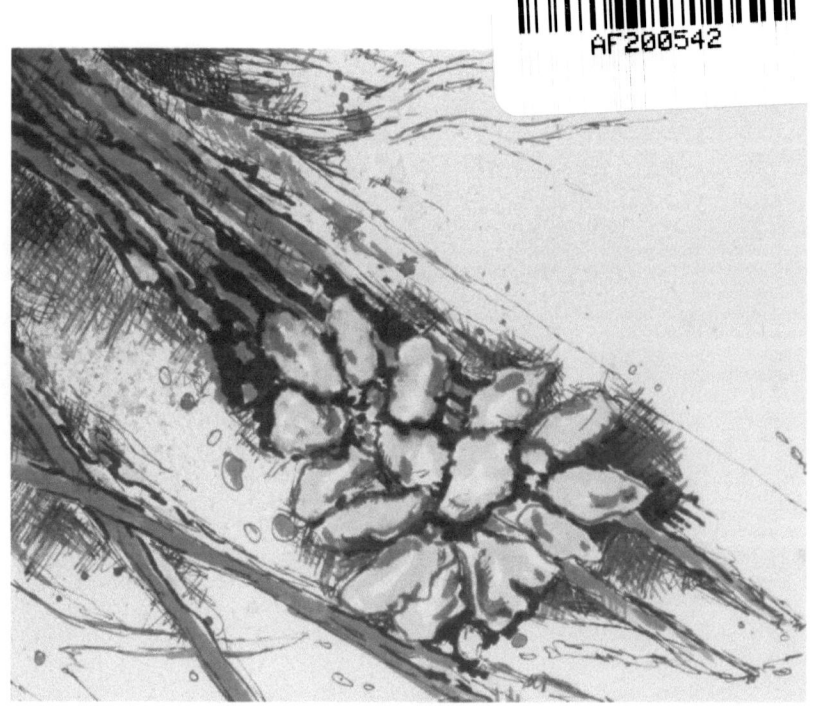

How it deceives medicine and makes us sick

- and how to diagnose and treat it

Editor's Note

This book was written by my friend, Dr. Uwe Auf der Straße.

Using an English alphabet, Auf der Straße would be written as Auf (of) der (the) Strasse (Street), and the 'Uwe' is pronounced Ooo-vah. Simple!

The book details how a family doctor in Germany made the connection between what he was seeing in his practice and a small piece of information which led him to 'follow the science' and uncover a connection between a parasite and debilitating symptoms, which had not been noted before. Probably other physicians had been presented with the same information, but Uwe's deductions represents the best of a marriage of scientific knowledge, intelligence, dogged persistence and an abiding desire to help his patients. It also shows how the General Practitioner, able to see the "wholeness" of the patient, may see patterns specialists don't see.

New ideas meet resistance, and Uwe has encountered entrenched ideas and has had to do much of the development of his treatments alone.

His dedication to his patients is wonderful and changes lives. Perhaps your life or the life of someone close to you will be one of those.

Bob Gougeon, MA

The case collection, on which the present book is based, as well as the book itself have been composed independently and without influence or financial contributions by companies or private persons. The case collection can be downloaded free of charge on toxoplasmachronic.com.

All statements in this book concerning the compromised sensitivity of the lab results when it comes to diagnosing Toxoplasma gondii should not be understood as criticism of medical labs. They surely do their work with utmost care, but most available tests are not suitable to detect bradyzoites and their activity. There is an urgent need to develop and refine such methods.

Caution: this book addresses a health-related topic. It is not supposed to replace consultation with a physician, nor is it meant to be used for self-diagnosis. The presented therapies are available only by prescription from a doctor. Self-treatment is strongly discouraged. All liability of the author for personal injury, property or financial damage will be declined.

Acknowledgements:

I would like, first and foremost, to thank my family for their loving patience and enthusiastic support. It is difficult to share a husband and father with a time-consuming profession, and this does not get any easier once he has started to write. I would also like to thank my wonderful parents, who have always encouraged me and who gave me the chance to study medicine.

My heartfelt thanks to my colleague Dr. med. J. Thiel and our entire surgery team. It is of great value to have an outstanding colleague and an excellent, committed team of employees at ones' side. And I wish to thank my patients. Without their confidence and openness in long conversations, some aspects of this disease would have remained hidden from me.

I would like to explicitly express my gratitude to Professor Jaroslav Flegr of Prague, Professor Vernon Carruthers of Michigan and Professor Robert Yolken of Baltimore for their scientific support. All three have been doing research in this field for many years and due to their ground breaking findings have contributed a lot to the understanding of Toxoplasma gondii. They have helped me tremendously with their scientific information and comments. I would also like to thank my highly valued colleague Dr. Hopf-Seidel for the exchange of experience.

Again, my special thanks go to Mrs. Andrea Thommes
for translation and
to my friend Bob Gougeon
for his excellent and indispensable proofreading
and advice

Cover: BoD   picture: *Bettina von Bichowski*

by Dr. med. U. Auf der Straße

Table of Contents

Preface

After 27 years of professional experience including 18 years of working as a general practitioner, quite some experience and insights with regards to the personal as well as the professional sphere have been accumulated. Especially for the interpersonal experiences I am very thankful to my patients. It is difficult to describe this. Most patients are warm-hearted and open minded, and often this helps us to get through the day. Most of them also deal with their illnesses in a wise and differentiated way and they are also increasingly better informed. It is surely a big mistake in medicine to underestimate patients too often.

On the professional side, one also never really stops learning. Only up to 30% of the GP's work is "coughing, sneezing and sore throat" cases that can be dealt with in a quick and clear way. By far the greater part of the work consists of intensive patient consultations and examinations to establish the correct diagnosis and to prescribe the right therapy. Frequent communication and more with a specialist colleague or a hospital is necessary. This diagnostic, therapeutic, supervisory and coordinating work of a GP is often underrated with regards to necessary knowledge as well as to the time required.

There are also unusual cases where things do not run smoothly, and these will be discussed here. The diagnosis sometimes does not explain all symptoms, the medication does not work as planned or is not tolerated, examinations perhaps do not help, and patients and doctor are discontent.

These are challenging cases, and only "staying on the ball", consistent reconsideration, talking with the patient, re-reading and re-examining may help advance a diagnosis.

Only in rare cases the symptoms are imaginary or the result of a somatic symptom disorder (more about this later) and even in unusual cases there is almost always an explanation, if only we can find it. A trusting cooperation between patient and doctor is indispensable. This includes that the doctor doesn't classify the symptoms of his patient as "psychosomatic" when the technical tests don't deliver conclusive results. Things don't work out without a certain amount of persistence, and sometimes there has to be worked again and again on a case for months, until a coherent and convincing diagnosis can be found.

If then the condition of the patient improves significantly, this makes the team simply happy and the finest job in the world is especially enjoyable then. In the search for conclusive answers and treatments for my patients, the parasite Toxoplasma gondii has proven to be a hard opponent. Its activity causes much more diseases than is generally assumed, and it is difficult to diagnose because it is equipped with a nearly perfect disguise.

All things considered, there *are* ways to diagnose it and to successfully treat this disease. Particularly the last 5 years have been a fine, strenuous and highly exciting time for me, which yielded significant findings for my work. Without the trust and good cooperation of my patients this would not have been possible.

> *Join me in the search for the code of this disease, the combination of symptoms, that reveal the activity of Toxoplasma gondii and thus make a decisive treatment possible. It is the most important and exciting chapter of my whole professional life, and it might be relevant to you as well.*

About this book

Until just 5 years ago, I did not suspect that the significance of Toxoplasma gondii (pronounced TOX-o-plaz-ma GON-dee-eye) for our health is extending far beyond what I learned in lecture hall HMA10 at Bochum University so many years ago, and that this parasite would one day play such an important role in my work. The idea of writing a paper or even a book about this topic would have seemed preposterous to me. It is generally assumed that toxoplasma cysts, which between 30 and 60% of the world population carry for a lifetime, are inactive and pose no risk whatsoever.

This is a major error, but that was my belief until I could diagnose one of my patients, who had been suffering for years from a severe unclear disease, with a chronic active toxoplasmosis. The appropriate Toxoplasma specific treatment was highly effective. This was a breakthrough, and she could return to her normal life and is healthy today.

I was startled, because along with my colleagues I did not consider active toxoplasmosis as a possible cause of disease in patients with intact immune system until this case happened. While working my way through the relevant medical literature and recent results of basic research I was amazed to find how extremely ingenious Toxoplasma gondii is in deceiving our immune system and our laboratory medicine. Unfortunately, some important research findings have not been transferred to applied (curative) medicine during the last 15 years.

Could it be possible that this parasite deceives us still and that far more people than previously assumed are chronically suffering from this disease?

The simple answer is "yes", and based on scientific evidence and presented in a clear and comprehensive language, I will explain how Toxoplasma gondii manages just that, why our laboratory results have largely failed so far, and how we can nevertheless detect and treat the disease that results when Toxoplasma increases its activity.

In Germany around 50% of the population or 41 million people are confirmed infected with this parasite. In the USA about 11% or approximately 40 million people are infected and worldwide about 30-60%, thus up to about 4 billion people. This is certainly too much for an "insignificant" parasite, and a significant number of people are taken ill because of it.

A specific form of this parasite cannot be identified by most of the currently available laboratory methods due to its almost perfect disguise, but precisely this form can be surprisingly active. This has been verified in several studies and has been known for about ten years, but medicine still relies heavily on laboratory results alone, and the symptoms of this disease are largely disregarded. Things are running smoothly for the parasite, because that way its activity takes place below our medical radar, and thus serious illnesses remain untreated.

The result is an often long-term clinical picture comprising chronic muscle pains, significantly reduced physical capacity, weariness, dyspnoea (shortness of breath after only light exercise), sweating, concentration disorders and much more. Unhelpful diagnoses such as "unclear myositis", "unclear cardiac insufficiency", "chronic fatigue from unknown cause", "fibromyalgia", "somatized depression" and many more are frequently observed.

As long as our laboratory results cannot safely detect a chronic active toxoplasmosis, it can only be revealed with difficulty.

> *Chronic active toxoplasmosis can be rightly described as a "shadow disease", not only acting stealthily in a kind of shadow, but also overshadowing the lives and stealing the health of those who suffer from it. The key to the detection of this disease is its combination of symptoms. Identifying this combination is the way the disease can be diagnosed, and this way will be precisely described in this book.*

Once it has been diagnosed, a chronic active toxoplasmosis can be treated effectively by any doctor using conventional allopathy drugs (allopathy just means commonly prescribed), and many people with hereto unclear clinical pictures could thus receive crucial help. This might be hard to believe, but due to the results of basic research and my own findings, I am deeply convinced that this is the plain truth.

I documented all these cases meticulously, thereby getting to know more of the diseases' symptoms with every case, and until now I have treated more than 150 patients successfully with the appropriate therapies. Twenty-seven of the first case documentations from the years 2015 to 2017 were compiled together with the corresponding scientific background in a paper. This book is based upon these results and the practical knowledge of the last five years. If we estimate only 25 patients with a Toxoplasma-related illness for every GP in Germany, the total will be about 800,000 persons affected, with considerably more probable, and it can be assumed that there are many more worldwide.

This book has been written in in order to be comprehensible for anyone interested in the subject. It also outlines the scientific and therapeutic foundations in such a detailed way that doctors can become acquainted with the topic and use it for their work. The chapters "work" widely independently, so that you might gain a first overview reading the chapters 1, 3, 6, 8 and 11, and hopefully feel then inclined to study the whole book.

If I had one free medical wish, it would be

that medicine could free itself from the outdated idea that these parasites were "harmless" and we had "a firm grip" on them. At the moment, the wind is entirely blowing the other way and a great many critically ill people, who are on an arduous odyssey through various medical institutions are in urgent need of an appropriate therapy.

If you are affected by this disease, this book may change your health for the better.

If you are healthy, you will read a thrilling and interesting book about a disease, which has been underrated again and again for 110 years and you will learn to be careful and watch out for Toxoplasma gondii.

If you are a doctor, please get yourself acquainted with the scientific fundamentals of this disease and analyse its symptoms. You might be able to help a lot of patients, but in doing so, please do not rely unconditionally on lab results, since they are still largely outsmarted by Toxoplasma.

In the last years, thanks to the diagnosis and therapy of Toxoplasma gondii, I have become able to help people with a disease that was out of my reach before.

The whole project started in 2014, with the treatment of the first patient, who had been suffering from an unclear illness for years and who recovered after the toxoplasmosis treatment. This is the case that will be presented in the next chapter.

1. This is not psychosomatic

In every practice there are some patients whose medical tests have not been completed or the preliminary diagnosis could not be verified, or the prescribed treatment may not help effectively. There are always some riddles and tricky courses of treatment that need to be deciphered. As a doctor, you have to face these situations and you must not give up under any circumstance or use the term "psychosomatic" as an easy way out. This might be arduous, but it is the only way. If you are a patient, you should not accept such a diagnosis without question.

It was the Autumn of 2014 and I was sitting with a patient in a quiet side room. The rest of the practice was buzzing with activity, but there and then I was exclusively focused on this patient. She reported, again, that until some 10 years ago she had been a very cheerful and fit person but that she had been suffering for at least 5 years from an unclear chronic fatigue, exhaustion and concentration disorder. She often failed to concentrate, made too many mistakes, and thus her work had become more and more arduous.

Within the last 2 years her health had deteriorated further. Dizziness and dyspnoea (shortness of breath) even while doing only minor physical work had developed. Examinations and laboratory tests had not yet yielded a decisive pointer, and so my expert colleagues and I had not found a satisfactory explanation for her illness. Thus, we had not been able to offer her an effective therapy.

"Why am I always so tired?", "Am I depressive?", "I can hardly take care of my children", "Why do I always hurt all over?" She had lots of questions, all of which were justified.

The young mother had been treated in hospital several times, also a mother-child rehabilitation had not yielded a tangible improvement. In the meanwhile, she had come to the conclusion that she was suffering from a psychosomatic disease.

> *In clinical pictures of psychosomatic illnesses, mental problems affect the physiological well-being so strongly that the mind ("psyche") makes the body ("soma") ill. Such clinical pictures have been increasing in Germany for years. No wonder, considered the pressure under which a lot of people live and work. In this context, psychotherapists trust medicine to have worked faultlessly and that no physical reasons for the clinical picture prevail.*
>
> *But "medicine" is by no means free from fault, just as there are no "infallible" doctors and psychotherapists. Unfortunately, for some years medicine has developed the unpleasant automatic response of a psychosomatic diagnosis if technical examinations deliver normal results. This also means that some doctors have unconditional trust in technology – only, why should technology be infallible?!*
>
> *The danger is that patients are downright "branded", and in my opinion, this is a real danger. Considering the constantly increasing number of psychosomatic cases I am afraid that psychosomatic diag-noses are sometimes made prematurely or, even worse, used as an easy way out.*

The patient now explained that her complaints were maybe "ima-ginary" and then in the same sentence she contradicted herself: "I am surely not going bonkers!" I shared this viewpoint with her, I really had not the impression that her complaints were "imaginary".

I felt the clinical picture was far too specific, too constant, and furthermore, the young woman assured me several times that apart from her disease she was generally leading a happy life. She couldn't recount psychologically stressful situations and traumatizing events, so how could her psyche then have caused such a severe illness?

Fate had it that in October 2014 I had to prescribe this patient an antibiotic for a severe infection. The infection improved, but to my surprise she also reported that her muscular pains had decreased significantly for the duration of the antibiotic treatment. This made me contemplate, "OK...if I have "side-treated" some "other" illness, what was that?!" Could there be a solution for this patient? I could investigate that an active toxoplasmosis could be able to trigger just the combination of symptoms from which the patient had been suffering, and that laboratory testing for this disease was not 100% reliable. I then initiated a further specialized examination in a neurological clinic, to make sure that the patient had not been suffering from a particular type of Borreliosis (Lyme's Disease. Read more on p.65)

After this had also been ruled out, the only remaining logical explanation for the clinical picture was Toxoplasmosis. The treatment for Toxoplasmosis has been known for a long time, and I prescribed the medication. Finally, a decisive improvement could be observed. Within just a few weeks, the therapy resulted in the recovery of the patient. If this happens in a case so severe, as a doctor you won't forget it! This has to be addressed as a contradiction because it is a kind of deeply engraved medical standard that in healthy persons without further health risks in their medical history, toxoplasmosis is supposed to trigger only light and temporary symptoms.

In the beginning I considered this case to be an unusual, fortunate single case – up until being faced with the next "single case" - and the next one... This obvious contradiction to accepted medicine required explanations, and I did my best to solve the riddle.

Our "opponent", Toxoplasma gondii, has been developing over the course of very long periods of time and is perfectly adapted to inhabiting us. Using its outstanding camouflage abilities, it plays a fascinating game of "cat and mouse" with our immune system and triggers severe illnesses in the afflicted, while our lab techniques tend to fail to reveal these activities.

The findings, which I could gather from this and all other treated cases, are mostly in accordance with previous medical findings and recent results of basic research, but I strongly disagree with my colleagues about the accuracy of the laboratory tests we currently rely on.

Particularly in terms of Toxoplasmosis it has been proven that lab results can be very unreliable and research also tells us why this is the case. Unfortunately, this has not led to changes in daily clinical work. The multiply possible symptoms of an active toxoplasmosis can be mistaken for a "psychosomatic" disease when a test erroneously indicates no active infection, but this is a serious major error that has to be avoided. We should listen to our patients, give credit to their descriptions, ask precisely for their symptoms and weigh them correctly because this disease can be identified and treated successfully, once it has been diagnosed.

2.   Several million years earlier

Evolution is in full swing and organisms are constantly looking for niches in which they may survive and reproduce, i.e. a place in the ecosystem. A tiny parasite, *Toxoplasma gondii* , a relative of malaria and only slightly bigger than a bacterium, starts to proliferate in a predator-prey loop. The life cycle of this creature is fascinating. The jackpot for this parasite is infecting a cat. Toxoplasma is not picky and every cat serves its purpose. If a cat has ingested Toxoplasma by eating infected prey, it falls ill. This usually takes place quite early in life, since cats are predators and many rodents and grazers are infected. Toxoplasma makes sure of that in a very effective way.

In the case of disease, sexual reproduction of Toxoplasma takes place inside the cat's gut, and only there. Sexual reproduction is evolution's model of success, because it enables the recombination of successful genes on a wide scale. If different Toxoplasma strains "meet" inside a cat, Toxoplasma can develop its genetic material by recombination (37), and that still happens today. After initial infection, the cat defecates large amounts of "oocysts", protective covers which contain the actual eggs, with its faeces for about 3 weeks. These are then widely spread throughout the cat's habitat.

Every oocyst then develops 8 infectious "sporozoites" in an inter-mediate stage within the next 2 days. The oocysts are very resistant even in a stressful environmental surrounding and can survive in the soil for up to several years. If it rains, they are spread by being washed away, and reach the surrounding plants and this way they get in contact with their next host in this chain. This is often the preferred prey of cats, but about 400 species have been found in which Toxoplasma can survive.

This includes all livestock kept by man, and a range of others up to anchovies and seals. Again, Toxoplasma is not picky. Inside these now infected "interim hosts", Toxoplasma cannot reproduce sexually (in contrast to the cat's gut), but its number still increases rapidly inside this interim host following the first days of infection by means of a special cell division, and they are then distributed throughout the whole organism of that host.

Then they are attacked by the host's immune system. Their strategy is to convert to a different form, and while doing so they change their surface structure nearly completely (75, 76). This is a major factor in the parasite's strategy of survival since the host's immune system, which identifies microorganisms according to their surface structure, is deceived successfully.

These other forms of Toxoplasma are called bradyzoites (brady: Greek for "slow") and they are specialized in evading the immune system for many years and yet can still reproduce effectively, especially when their host is affected by other diseases. Their role extends far beyond mere survival. In fact, they prepare their host over years to become a more suitable prey for cats by becoming saturated with cysts and significantly weakened.

This activity gradually leads to permanent exhaustion, muscles hurt increasingly and cardiovascular capacity decreases significantly. Finally, concentration and visual capacity of the host are impaired. Several years later, the victim contains ample numbers of bradyzoites and is considerably weakened, so that is becomes an ideal prey. Often, the prey victim is then devoured by a cat and thus the circle is complete.

So, we and all of our livestock are intermediate hosts and are simply used as "carriers", which over the years get saturated with bradyzoite cysts, until they are then put to final "use" by Toxoplasma. This ingenious system has been misunderstood by research in former times. It was believed that the parasites inside us would be passive and inactive. In fact, the whole process of changing the appearance and building up intracellular cysts is nothing but a skilful adjustment of tactics to avoid a direct battle with our immune system.

> But by no means do the parasites give up their biological program while doing so. In order to infect a cat, they will still use any chance to multiply (42, 84), weaken the host and influence its behaviour (see pp. 49 - 50, 169 - 183). Our health is obviously no concern to the parasites.

> It is remarkable that the parasite does not only significantly increase the probability of being eaten by a cat through a severe physical weakening of the host, but also through a significant decrease of its mental capacity. Toxoplasma also modifies the hosts' behaviour to its own favour. We cannot assume Toxoplasma to be intelligent, but still it acts extremely skilfully, and over years it reduces the quality of life and the host's survivability significantly. This entire system has been perfected over very long periods of time, and we are still being prey in a biological sense, only we are too blind to see this. It is about time that we take note of this fact.

> "Toxoplasmosis is a chronic global disease that burdens human beings and animals" (40).

3. Algeria 1909, Prague 1923, New York 1938, Palo Alto 1994, Wolverhampton 2003, Sao Paulo 2006

Algeria 1909

At Institut Pasteur in Tunis, where today vaccines are still produced, doctors Nicolle and Manceaux discovered Toxoplasma gondii in 1909.
"The" instrument in research is the optical microscope and microscopical examinations were carried out quite naturally by many doctors then. Within the framework of their research, they examined a perished "gundi" (a small African rodent of guinea pig-size). In the tissue samples they found strange comma-shaped microorganisms which form cysts inside the tissue and which do not act like bacteria at all. They classified their recovery as protoplasma (small, single-cell organisms) and named them "Toxoplasma gondii", which means "curvilinear organism in gondi". They publish an article with the title *"Sur un protozoario noveau du gondii"* about this finding in a renowned professional journal (61). Since other colleagues also carry out microscopical examinations, Toxoplasma will be identified several times in connection with cases of illness in human in the following years and the diseases resulting from this are recorded.

Prague 1923, Czech Children's Hospital

The ophthalmologist Josef Janků described the sad case of a child, who died at the age of 11 months. It had been suffering from "hydrocephalus", a congenital deformation. This translates to "brain filled with water", a sadly fitting expression, since it describes a circulation disorder of the cerebral fluid that results in a swelling of the whole head. In the *fundus oculi* (the interior of the eye) clear signs of toxoplasmosis were found.

This is considered to be the first proven case of toxoplasmosis-induced illness in humans. This physician also succeeded in taking the first photograph of Toxoplasma. As we know today, hydrocephalus may develop as a result of infection with Toxoplasma gondii in the maternal womb. Janků, 1923 (47)

New York 1938, Babies' Hospital

On 23ʳᵈ May 1938, a little girl was born.   She was ill and as early as 3 days after birth a retinal inflammation of both eyes developed. The girl sadly died just one month later. Toxoplasma gondii was found in lesions of encephalomyelitis and retinitis (inflammations of the brain and retina) of the girl. With these samples it is also proven that Toxoplasma gondii can be transferred to laboratory animals. This is probably the first indication that there is no biological barrier between animals and humans for this parasite.   Wolf et al. 1938 (89).

Palo Alto, California, November 1994

A 43-year old woman with a life-threatening cardiac insufficiency was admitted into the communal hospital suffering from undefined muscular pains and headaches. Furthermore, the GP noted a singular lymph node swelling and flu-like symptoms. Prior to this illness, she had been very resilient. Mountain hikes with gradients of up to 45° for a distance of approximately 2 miles were accomplished without problem. A Heart catheter examination showed unconstricted coronary vessels, but the cardiac ejection fraction (the amount of blood pumped) was decreased down to 30%.

A tissue sample from the cardiac muscle revealed an inflammation of the myocardium (tissue surrounding the heart). With the help of laboratory examinations, an acute toxoplasmosis was diagnosed as reason for the muscular pains, headaches and myocarditis. In the course of the progression, an additional inflammation of the retina developed. The patient had very probably been infected with toxoplasmosis when eating uncooked lamb 4 weeks before. After repeated toxoplasmosis treatments the patient recovered from the disease.

This is an exceptionally well documented case, which can only be reported in a very abbreviated version here. The original is particularly worth reading for doctors. As a consequence, the attending doctors recommend that toxoplasmosis should be considered in cases of unexplained inflammation of the cardiac muscle or muscles in general. Montoya, 1997 (58).

Wolverhampton Primary Care Trust, England, 2003

Doctors were racking their brains why a 32-year old man seemed to be slipping more and more into a severe depression. They examined him again thoroughly and it became apparent that along with this depression, he has been suffering from further symptoms for seven months, including pronounced general weakness, dizziness and tinnitus. Further technical examinations showed an increased rate of Toxoplasma antibodies, but no other conspicuous findings were made. The doctors thus started a therapy against toxoplasmosis and could finally note a significant improvement. Also, the antidepressants started to work then and the patient recovered completely within 6 months. Nilamadhab Kar & Baikunthanath Misra 2003, (62)

A 41-year old man was admitted to the Emergency Department of Hospital do Servidor Público Estadual in São Paulo. The patient was healthy before and had not taken any medication. He had suffered from fever, headaches and muscular pains for 8 days, and for 4 days he suffered from nausea and vomiting. *Twenty days before he had eaten half-cooked meat.*

On examination, high fever and jaundice of unknown origin were noticed, as was an enlargement of the liver and spleen, as well as a significantly increased heart-rate of 115 beats per minute, but no swelling of the lymph nodes.

Liver enzyme readings and bilirubin were increased, which is a typical finding for jaundice. Further laboratory values were found, which remained inexplicable at first. Thirty-six hours after admission, a double-sided pneumonia occurred and the condition of the patient worsened dramatically. A decrease of oxygen concentration in the blood pointed towards an imminent risk, and the attending doctors decided to start an oxygen therapy and administered infusions with a combination of 3 antibiotics. This also didn't help and further blood tests were undertaken which showed positive results for Toxoplasma antibodies. A combination therapy against toxoplasmosis was started at once.

In the following 3 days, the patient's pulmonary situation deteriorated further and a severe anaemia developed. From the fourth day of the toxoplasmosis therapy onwards a significant improvement occurred and to the great relief of all parties involved, the patient was discharged after a 12-day stay in hospital.

The toxoplasmosis therapy was continued for 30 days altogether. It was finally proven that Toxoplasma of the dangerous "type III" was involved, and it is surely remarkable how fast and aggressive the course of disease was, despite the patient being healthy before and not weakened by previous diseases. Without any doubt, the toxoplasmosis therapy was lifesaving here. Leal, Fabio Eudes et al. (54)

These are historic cases and some case reports from recent times. They all share that they describe acute progressions, and especially due to positive test results, toxoplasmosis could be treated successfully in the last 3 cases.

But still, the roots of the problem reach much deeper. Chronic cases of active toxoplasmosis can cause similar severe illnesses in the long run and affect many more people than hitherto assumed, but cannot be detected reliably with the help of laboratory tests alone. I will explain in detail, which symptoms are to be expected, why laboratory values alone are not reliable enough to identify these cases securely, how the disease progresses, how it can be treated, and why medicine does not yet decisively diagnose it.

4. A living microcosm

We now need to have a closer look at microorganisms. Evolution takes place on many different levels at the same time, and the survival of one species is not only determined by how strongly and quickly (and possibly intelligently) the individuals can act. There is also a microscopic level, where real battles are fought. We also profit from these altercations. Our immune system would not likely have become as effective as it is, had it not be forced to continuously deal with microorganisms and also to partially cooperate with them.

This goes as far as living in a *symbiotic relationship* with many of these microorganisms. It means that both parties, the microorganisms, which can survive on and inside us and we human beings can profit. Our immune system is trained, and in the case of intestinal bacteria it has been proven that our immune system's competence, i.e. the recognition of friend and foe, only results from a close cooperation with these bacteria.

Bacteria also keep each other in check, so we are involved with an ecosystem that can keep up its own equilibrium. Our immune system's task is it to supervise and to correct dangerous deviations. I am convinced that basic research about the relations among these microorganism as well as research about relations about our body and immune system have the potential to develop medicine significantly in coming years.

Unfortunately, some microorganisms are "egoistic", and this can result in *parasitic relationships* between organisms. One organism, usually much bigger than the other, is the host, whose well-being and survivability is impaired. The other organism, e.g. Toxoplasma gondii, is the parasite, which burdens the host in a one-sided way and profits from him, sometimes with deadly consequences.

5. Parasites

Parasites take a one-sided benefit from their hosts, and being free-loaders, they do not enjoy a high reputation. I have to admit that I shared that point of view during my studies. This life principle seems to be quite successful, and it is assumed that the majority of organisms on our planet lead a parasitic existence. In comparison to viruses and bacteria, parasites exhibit different dynamics. Their strategy is usually slow, careful and sustainable for their own benefit. Initially they mostly trigger only chronic symptoms, but the progression can also be lethal. To avoid a direct battle with the host's immune system they are often well-camouflaged, and this can result in difficulties diagnosing them.

It is generally not a parasite's aim to overrun the host and to eventually (too quickly) kill him in the process, but rather to assure an effective reproduction of its own species. Weakening the host is a frequent side-effect, but his life is not threatened yet. Parasites mostly inhabit their hosts for longer periods of time, and who wants to burn down his own house? There is furthermore abundant evidence to prove that parasites can trigger behavioural changes in host organisms (and that means us! see pp. 175 - 179). From a parasite's point of view this is highly sensible, from the host's point of view it is not. That is because a parasite has its own agenda and once we have served our cause, it is no longer interested in our survival...

Illnesses caused by parasites often persist for several years and mostly progress slower and less dramatically than acute illnesses. Therefore, they are mostly "chronic" and there are effective drugs against many parasites. This has unfortunately led to the widespread belief, even among doctors, that these diseases were under control.

Unfortunately, slowly developing chronic diseases tend to act below our medical "radar" and, if we do not take *every symptom* of into account, we can misdiagnose a disease, as our medicine is strongly focused on acute diseases and technically methods. All in all, this is not a bad environment for parasites, since they are masters of camouflage and they often cannot be detected accurately, despite the use of highly developed technology. As a result, parasitology as a medical discipline is regarded as being a rather "small" field, which bears little relevance for daily medicine.

Not recognizing the cause of symptoms might then lead to the conclusion that some "psychosomatic" problem causes the disease. *This is a major error.* In terms of diagnostics, we almost exclusively rely on lab diagnostics, which we expect will deliver "perfect" results – but is this realistic?

This leads us back to *Toxoplasma gondii*, a parasite, whose biological program is so particularly refined that it has been mocking medicine until today. With a perfect camouflage, it can adapt to many different hosts and it is able to "flood" the host organism with a high rate of reproduction in the face of a weakened immune system. Nevertheless, when being attacked by the host´s immune system, it can also retreat into the cells quickly, change its appearance, reproduce in protected cavities and survive there for a lifetime. The disease that results from Toxoplasma activity is described on pages 49 -51.

Toxoplasma is capable of so much more and are therefore is a very tough and difficult opponent for the host organism. Its excellent camouflage makes it very difficult to be kept in check by our immune system in the long-term, and compromises the reliability of our lab methods seriously. The next chapter will present some of its secrets - but I am sure there will be unveiled even more in the future.

5. Toxoplasma gondii – a master of disguise

Toxoplasma gondii is a single-celled parasite and only slightly bigger than bacteria. Several hundred of it fit inside single muscle cells or neurons, *and there are almost no restrictions for them*. As far as known, it can infect all warm-blooded creatures, and Toxoplasma have even been found in fishes and sea mammals. According to recent knowledge, about 30%-60% of the world's population carry Toxoplasma gondii (64). This is about 2 to 4 billion people, but even in 2019, 110 years after the discovery of Toxoplasma, the effects and consequences of this infestation have not fully been understood.

In comparison, "only" little more than 1 billion people worldwide are infected with malaria, a related parasitic tropical disease (Bundesgesundheitsblatt 2008 / 51: 236-249). Malaria relies on the Anopheles mosquito as "key factor" and is therefore restricted more to the tropics and sub-tropics. By using cats as a means of reproduction and distribution, Toxoplasma gondii is less climate-sensitive, and toxoplasma are found all over the world. From this point of view, Toxoplasma gondii is even "more successful" than malaria.

Today we are looking back on 110 years of research on toxoplasmosis, which have given us thorough and detailed insights. Those doctors and scientists who have gifted us with this recent standard of knowledge deserve our thanks and respect. However, toxoplasma are masters of disguise and have been blinding doctors and researchers about their dangerous potential by means of their sophisticated mechanisms of camouflage and deception until today. Findings, which could correct this, have been known for some years, but have hardly affected the field outside a small group of scientists.

We now have to amalgamate this knowledge urgently and make use of it for the benefit of our patients, because Toxoplasma activity results in many more cases than we have assumed (31) see also p. 165.

The reproduction of Toxoplasma gondii works like this. Toxoplasma survive the passage through stomach and gut in oocysts (eggs) or also in bradyzoites (in infected meat). Inside the host, they quickly transform into "tachyzoites". This initially occurring, "fast" form of Toxoplasma can trigger severe, acute pictures of disease and have thus been the focus of research for many years.

They can move very effectively and are able to invade quickly, within a few seconds, nearly any cell. There they create temporary caverns (pseudocysts) and reproduce with a specific type of cell-division until they number several hundred per cell. These cells burst and release new tachyzoites. Speed is absolutely of the essence then, since the host's immune system has already identified the attacker and starts to produce antibodies in great quantities. These antibodies are specifically tailored towards attacking viruses, bacteria or parasites, and are destined to dock with their surface structures and thus mark them as prey for huge white immune cells, called "macrophages".

The available antibody tests only record those antibodies specific to tachyzoites.

A first catch is that research findings as early as 1964 presented at the First International Congress for Parasitology showed that not all laboratory animals infected with Toxoplasma developed detectable antibodies (48), and this was confirmed later (24, 53).

It is still unknown today how many people do not develop detectable antibodies after an infection with Toxoplasma. A test for antibodies in these people would not show the presence of Toxoplasma.

Our immune system's preparations for defence take about one week and during that time Toxoplasma reproduces and try to spread as far as possible. The parasite prefers neural and muscular tissue, but can also invade other organs. Apart from solid bones there is nothing that they cannot reach.

So, the week is over ....and now they will be taken under fire, right...?

No, not really, since it has been common knowledge since 1976 that the antibodies we produce, offer only very little protection against Toxoplasma (32). The reason why this is the case was found a lot later. It had been known that Toxoplasma change into a different form, bradyzoites, due to the immune system's increasing pressure. But it was only discovered in 1996 that in doing so they change the surface structure of their outer membrane to a great extent (76, 77). This is a brilliant biological camouflage, which gives toxoplasma a crucial advantage, because it is highly probable that antibodies cannot dock to the bradyzoites due to this structural change.

To make sure that Toxoplasma, now in the form of bradyzoites, is really safe from the immune system and that this won't start a production of bradyzoite specific antibodies, the parasites now invade the host cell deeply.

They take over parts of the "interior" of their host cells, from which they create solid, durable cysts. These cysts will be their home for many years to come. Here, they are protected and can power down their metabolism. In this form, they induce nearly no bradyzoite specific antibody production (95), so their hiding place is very effective.

The lab tests currently in use do not detect bradyzoites themselves or bradyzoite antibodies.

On the other hand, bradyzoites can still reproduce, especially if the host's immune system is not attentive enough, weakened (6, 42) or over-burdened by other disease factors. It has been known for a long time that inside these cysts, Toxoplasma can survive and remain infectious within a host for a lifetime, but it was assumed that in this form they would be "passive" and "inactive" and thus no threat to the host-organism.

However, it is now known that even after their transformation from tachyzoites to bradyzoites, Toxoplasma are significantly more active than assumed earlier. First hints reach back to 1989 (26). In 2008 an extensive study was published which focused on the *long-term effect* of an active toxoplasmosis (42). In neuronal tissue of infected mice there were found signs of inflammation, structural damage of the tissue and a lot of bradyzoite cysts, which together resulted in a seriously impaired health and altered behaviour of the mice.

The researchers could also show that bradyzoites are able to evoke this disease on their own, without the "support" of tachyzoites.

It is also known that bradyzoite - activity as well as tachyzoite - activity can induce increased cytokines in atrocytes and microglial cells (specialized immune cells of the brain (27)), and cytokines are known to induce inflammation and depression (see literature reference on page 177). In 2015 another proof of activity of bradyzoites was found by a team of researchers at the University of Kentucky (84). Researchers could establish in animal testing that new bradyzoite cysts can be formed in the course of a chronic toxoplasmosis and concluded that bradyzoites can cause chronic diseases. Particularly cells of the muscular and nerve tissue can be filled with several hundreds of bradyzoites after a number of years.

All this considered, bradyzoites are surely not "harmless".

The antibodies, which are produced by our immune system with great effort are tailored exclusively to the "fast" form of Toxoplasma, the tachyzoites, and are only effective against them. They cannot reach the "slow" types, i.e. the bradyzoites in their cysts, and they most likely couldn't "dock" to them anyhow, because of their changed surface structure.

After their change to bradyzoites, Toxoplasma can therefore only be kept in check by our immune system with great difficulty. At that point, the Toxoplasma have retreated effectively and the immune system's hunt is temporarily ended. But in the form of bradyzoites, Toxoplasma have by no means entered a "cul-de-sac", as medicine has assumed for many years, because this life form only represents a clever change in tactics – and they are also not inactive, but rather hustle along the progression of the disease.

The knowledge that bradyzoites can be very active and a threat to health (26, 42, 84) has unfortunately not been adapted from scientific research to clinical medicine. Here, standard thinking still persists that bradyzoites are "harmless" and that our laboratory findings represent the disease process correctly.

According to basic research both assumptions are outdated, but they persist, and the result is that Toxoplasma related diseases are being excluded from diagnosis when lab tests show negative results. The ingenuity of Toxoplasma goes even further. They possess astounding skills, which help them to overcome another line of defence of our immune system, as will be described in the following. Our immune system does not master Toxoplasma. It can at best achieve a stalemate.

It has been known since 1989 that Bradyzoites can re-transform to their attacking form, i.e. the fast tachyzoites (26). Both shapes live together in the cysts, but under pressure of a healthy immune system there is a clear weighting towards bradyzoites. Several studies (6, 35, 78, 79) have proven that continuous activity of certain white blood cells is necessary to prevent Toxoplasma from becoming more active and to prevent them to break free from their cysts.

To achieve this, the white blood cells, especially CD8 cells, are constantly producing 4 different interferons, which are highly active messengers of the immune system. If the immune system is weakened considerably after a long course of a disease, these CD8 cells can lose their ability to produce two of these interferons. This was discovered by Badhra and Khan in 2012 (6).

They described this as an exhaustion of the CD8 cells, which in itself triggers a weakening of the immune system. This enables Toxoplasma to change into a more active stage of the disease.

> To the extent in which the exhaustion of the immune system progresses, more bradyzoites transform back to their tachyzoite shape. In case of a weakening immune system, the "army" thus gets ready to spread further within the organism. It is conceivable that while doing this, Toxoplasma sometimes is "aided" by other microorganisms, since the CD8 system can also be burdened, or especially in case of a combined attack, be overwhelmed by other pathogens.

Toxoplasma gondii is even able to survive in specialised immune cells, the "macrophages". These macrophages are particularly lethal for average invaders – but not for Toxoplasma. In order to kill pathogens, macrophages first assimilate and enfold them and fuse these cysts with "lysosomes", cellular components of the large white cell macrophages, which contain a lethal cocktail for microorganisms.

This fusion is prevented by Toxoplasma and thus renders the infected macrophages helpless. The hunter becomes the prey (19) as Toxoplasma can then reproduce inside the macrophages and make use of them as a Trojan horse, getting transported through the whole organism and thus entering the central nervous system (15).

Unfortunately, there is even more bad news. Toxoplasma can intervene and control our immune system. This has been known for some years now, and several studies about this have been published (3, 19, 76).

These are the reasons why Toxoplasma even in form of the presumed "harmless" bradyzoites can have such a severe impact on our health. Our immune system is not able eradicate toxoplasma completely, and it also doesn't master them, so it is rather a stalemate situation - but only as long as our immune system is strong enough to keep this situation in check. We have to live with them, once we have them on board.

Summarised, there are many reasons why Toxoplasma gondii can cause diseases in otherwise healthy humans who possess a fully intact immune system (i.e. "immunocompetent" people).   It has indeed already been found as early as 1974 that immunocompetent patients can suffer from toxoplasmosis (70) and in 1975 a study revealed that about half of the patients suffering from a cerebral inflammation due to Toxoplasma were immunocompetent (83).   In another study done in 1985, only 48 of 200 patients were rated immunocompetent (55), and from 1998 to 2006, 44 immunocompetent patients in French Guinea, whose case histories have been recorded meticulously, were suffering from toxoplasmosis (11).

So at least since 1974 several research results have been available to prove that a healthy immune system can be conquered by Toxoplasma., and it has also revealed how they achieve this. Since 1996, we know about the structural change of Toxoplasma´s surface during the transformation from tachyzoites to bradyzoites (77), which renders our antibodies inefficient towards bradyzoites and causes our laboratory findings, which search for those antibodies, to lose a lot of their accuracy.

Nevertheless, the same bradyzoites can be surprisingly active, cause inflammation (27) and tissue damage (42) and multiply (84). They can exhaust our immune system (6), and transform back to their "attacking state", the tachyzoite (25). If the immune system starts to work again more effectively at times, Toxoplasma is forced to reduce its activity and revert back to its bradyzoite state (25), but unfortunately this success is often not permanent.

This whole process then possibly leads to more and more bradyzoite cysts over the years, until the host is weakened and literally "saturated" with cysts, inside which the bradyzoites can multiply further.

It is hard to believe, but true, that all these findings don't play a major role in medicine today. They have not been widely noticed in scientific discussions, and did not lead, until today, to a re-thinking of the role of bradyzoites, which would be urgently needed. Toxoplasma act quite ingeniously, their strategy is clever and long-term and they are highly underestimated, especially in their bradyzoite form.

The bradyzoites' slowness and ostensible inertia have misled researchers to mistake them for years as being harmless. The laboratory methods we currently use, can not determine the "Toxoplasma load" we are carrying inside our bodies, and due to Toxoplasma's brilliant camouflage they also can not reveal bradyzoite activity. The parasites hold by far the better position, and we are making a huge mistake by still underestimating them.

The "trick" is the combination of errors. Some researchers know that the test systems are unable to detect bradyzoites, but don't recognize this as a problem, since the majority of researchers still consider bradyzoites to be inactive and harmless. Only very few of those researchers who point out an enhanced bradyzoite activity are working directly "on the patient".

Doctors in hospitals and GP's however are faced with patients who are suffering from symptoms of an active toxoplasmosis, but as a rule they are not aware that patients with a healthy immune system can indeed suffer from an active toxoplasmosis and that this disease cannot be detected by antibody test, if they are caused by bradyzoite activity.

The whole complex is a veritable Gordian knot. Since the problem is not recognized, there is no problem, and the error is no error. This is a catastrophe for the affected patients, because if their laboratory findings are negative, they might be then classified as "psycho-somatic". They won't get rid of this label easily. New test methods which can detect bradyzoite activity reliably could solve this problem but are still being developed (see from pp 209), and it might take years, until they are all validated (their reliability being proven by studies) and available.

This is a challenging situation, but we are anything but helpless. We can treat an active toxoplasmosis with powerful medication and even heal patients, once we have identified Toxoplasma activity as cause of a disease. Still, there is more basic information to be covered until we come to this point.

6.1. Modes of transmission

An infection can be caused by oocysts (protective capsules that contain Toxoplasma "eggs"), as well as by meat from infected animals that contains bradyzoite cysts. A human-to-human transmission can take place, when a woman undergoes an *initial* infection during pregnancy, where the infection can be passed on to the baby. A transmission of Toxoplasma is also possible if an organ donor is infected.

Cats mostly fall ill from toxoplasmosis at an age of a few weeks and then excrete a large number of oocysts with their faeces for about three weeks. These become infectious after about 2 days, once the sporozoites (the real "eggs") have been developed fully inside them. With the faeces, the oocysts with the contained sporozoites are distributed throughout the entire habitat of the cat, thus also in the garden, in the vegetable patch or in the sandbox. In the course of renewed Toxoplasma infections at a later stage, cats don't excrete oocysts in about 90% of the cases, since they develop a certain immunity (33).

The risk of infection due to direct contact with an infected cat might be reduced in older cats as they excrete fewer oocysts to their environment. But all together, contamination of soil with oocysts due to cat's faeces is a serious health hazard.

In 2013 a study on this topic was published (82). In the USA, about 1.2 million tons of cat's faeces per year in urban sectors (also in domestic gardens and in playgrounds!) lead to a measurable burden of 3 to 434 oocysts per square foot. To my knowledge, a corresponding research has not been done in Germany, but it would surely be misguided optimism to expect a lower contamination.

As a reminder, oocysts are very environmentally resistant and remain infectious for several years also on the pasture, in the field, in the garden or in the sandbox. A single oocyst, that finds its way inside the host organism by means of direct contact or on plant matter is sufficient to cause an infection of the human or the livestock and the human then becomes a life - long carrier of toxoplasma, and the meat of the livestock gets infectious.

This means of transmission is obviously very effective, since an infection of humans with Toxoplasma gondii is caused most frequently by bradyzoite cysts, which can be contained in uncooked meat from any livestock (14). Vegetarians are exposed to a slightly lower risk, but not everybody is willing to change his or her diet so fundamentally, and oocysts can also be ingested with vegetables that have not been washed thoroughly or with contaminated water (4). In effect, a Toxoplasma infection is a worldwide and lifelong risk.

6.2. The risk of infection can be reduced

The contact with infected cats should be avoided or reduced and the litter box of infected cats should be cleaned daily, before the oocysts have matured, which takes 2 days. Protective gloves should be worn in the process and a strict use of hand-hygiene is advisable. It is probably unavoidable that in a phase of acute toxoplasmosis in cats, oocysts also get stuck in the cat's fur and can thus be transmitted to human hands. *Thus, it is also advisable not to seek close physical contact to an ill cat. This applies particularly to children! Again, a strict hand-hygiene is to be observed at all times.*

It would probably be beneficial to keep cats away from and out of stables. This is most likely possible in factory farming, but I most certainly don't see this type of farming as desirable. Cats should be kept away from sandboxes *(which should be covered at all times)* and, if possible, also from vegetable patches. Gardening work should be done wearing protective gloves and hands should be cleaned thoroughly afterwards. As a general rule, lettuce should only be consumed after intensive washing. Wearing of protective gloves and frequent, and intensive washing of hands is to be observed when preparing meat and uncooked meat should not be sampled.

Beware: uncooked meat, e.g. a succulent steak done "medium" can certainly still contain viable Toxoplasma. Meat products should therefore rather be consumed well-done. An internal temperature of 67 °C, or 152 °F for ten minutes will kill Toxoplasma.

Another option to effectively kill bradyzoites in meat is a preliminary freeze, as research in 1991 has shown (52) Toxoplasma cysts are able to survive a temperature of -6.7°C for about 11 days. Below -12.2°C (9° F) no living bradyzoites can be detected after 8.5 hours. The freezing time in the domestic freezer has to be significantly longer for safety reasons, if the meat has not been frozen beforehand, since a temperature of -12.2°C (9° F) for at least 8.5 hours has to be achieved inside the frozen meat. Frozen food is stored at -18°C (0°F) in Germany and the US and can thus be considered safe (please check the guidelines for frozen food in your country).

It might be of increasing significance that there are different Toxoplasma strains, since it has been proven in 2011 that these strains can cross if they are found in one cat at the same time. New atypical variants might develop which could be even more dangerous than the known strains (38). This has initially been found in Southern European cats, but has also been found in German cats as early as 2010 (43, 72). This means that there could be significantly more aggressive strains of Toxoplasma in Germany and we should be better prepared. Still, the possible development of more aggressive strains might happen worldwide.

Beyond the risks of chronic active toxoplasmosis, the documented cases of acute toxoplasmosis presented on pages 24 - 28 give proof how dangerous and aggressive the resulting disease can be. We need urgently to prepare and also learn to protect ourselves better from Toxoplasma infections.

6.3   30-60% of the world population are infected

The estimated Toxoplasma infections of humans (59, 63) represent more the lower end. If some studies performed with animals are taken in account (24, 48, 53), it is reasonable that more humans are infected than lab results indicate.   There is proof that in some animals, for example pigs, there are infected individuals which exhibit no detectable antibodies. Corresponding research for humans has not yet been performed.

For the world population, a frequency of positive Toxoplasma assay of 30% has been estimated (59), with a variability of 10-60% (63).   This would be 2 to 4 billion people. There are some catches that explain why the presumed range is so huge.

The frequency of positive Toxoplasma IgG assays, which are mostly tachyzoite – specific assays, is known with some limitations, but the **error rate** for IgG assays in primary infections with a frequently used test system is approximately 18% (66), and this varies from test to test. (IgG assays search for a specific serum Immunoglobulin G produced by the immune system).   It is not known how long Toxoplasma IgG are detectable after a primary infection, so some years after this infection took place, there might be no detectable IgG anymore – although the infection might still persist.   A bradyzoite detection can, with some difficulties, only be performed in highly specialized labs and cannot be done in "normal" medical labs.

The rate of infection for women of childbearing age or pregnant women has been documented for many countries (64). On a world map, Germany, along with Belgium and France is highlighted as an area with high infection rates. Infection rates in North America (except Quebec) and Northern Europe are significantly lower at 11-20%.

In the Netherlands it was 26% in 2007 and probably the lowest rate was found in Thailand at about 5%. The rate of infection in the respective total population is probably higher, since the frequency of an infection with Toxoplasma increases with age (and especially older women are often disregarded in statistics), and the risk to men is often not recorded, as it is pregnant women who are tested.

In Germany, which may serve as an example for a high-risk area, frequency for positive Toxoplasma detection is about 50% of the adult population (88). Here, the frequency of positive Toxoplasma detection increases from about 20% in the group of 18-29 year-olds, up to 77% in the group of 70-79 year-olds and for over 79 year-olds the frequency is 84%. It is evident that the parasite simply has more time to "catch" us in the course of a longer lifetime. Eventually, Toxoplasma is ingested by means of a rare steak, other undercooked meat products or just unwashed lettuce. Toxoplasma is patient...

For men, the risk in comparison to women, is increased 1.76 times, a near doubling. Keeping of cats and already being slightly overweight with a BMI (Body Mass Index) above 30 are further risk factors. A vegetarian diet reduces the risk. In the East of Germany, the frequency in all age groups is significantly higher than in the West of Germany. In the group of 40-69 year-olds the difference amounts to 20%.

Due to the camouflage abilities of Toxoplasma gondii and the lack of precision of the currently used lab techniques it is challenging to estimate precise infection rates. Probably rates are higher than we have assumed, and there is no doubt that the possibility of getting infected with Toxoplasma gondii is a lifetime risk all over the world.

6.4. Symptoms of an active toxoplasmosis

Historically, various symptoms have been determined in connection with toxoplasmosis, and this makes diagnosing it so difficult. The possible symptoms are numerous, but not all of them are found at all times, and they can sometimes also be caused by other diseases. There is a way through the thick of this forest of symptoms, and it starts with scientific basics:

Muscular pain is a frequent symptom of an acutely acquired or reactivated toxoplasmosis (16, 37, 58). Behan et al. reported in 1983 a child with congenital toxoplasmosis as the source for a **combined inflammation of the skin and muscles** (7).

The heart muscle can also be affected. Montoya et al. reported in 1997 about a hitherto healthy, immunocompetent patient who developed an **inflammation of the cardiac muscle** with resulting severe **cardiac insufficiency** due to an active toxoplasmosis (58).

Pulmonary disease (11) and **involvement of the diaphragm** (an important muscle needed for breathing) were shown (53). These factors plus cardiac inflammation could individually or in combination result in a significant decrease in cardiac / pulmonary output, causing a severe **dyspnoea** (shortness of breath) under stress as a result.

Pressing sensations and sometimes pain in the upper and middle abdomen have been reported repeatedly. As a possible source, a Toxoplasma-related **liver infection** (23), an **inflammation of the abdominal lymph nodes** (51) and a Toxoplasma-related **stomach infection** (34) have already been described.

An inflammation of the **prostate** is also possible (13), which results in inflammation and frequent urination that resembles a bladder irritation. (compare symptoms of case 25, p. 150)

The preferred target tissue of the parasite apart from muscle tissue is the **central nervous system**, with **inflammations of the brain** and the **eyes** as a result (85). This is probably mediated by cytokines (27), which can be set free by tachyzoite- as well as bradyzoite-activity.

The ability to concentrate, the ability to think clearly and mental resilience can be severely affected by toxoplasmosis. In 2001 it was ascertained, that the reaction time in infected patients was significantly prolonged, and it progressed with increasing duration of infection. The researchers concluded that there is a slowly increasing, damaging effect of toxoplasmosis on humans' cognitive ability (39).

With the **cerebellum,** an important area for motor coordination, fine control and the learning of movement patterns can be affected, which causes **dizziness and unsteady gait** (37) as well as movements which are less precise and coordinated. Prof. Flegr from Prague proved in 2007 that a positive Toxoplasma assay increases the risk for causing a traffic accident by a factor of 2.6 (28).

Significant psychic changes in patients with a positive Toxoplasma assay included **aggressive behaviour, increased impulsiveness** (12), **more frequent occurrence of schizophrenia** (22, 81, 92), as well as **more frequent occurrence of anxieties, headaches, reduced intelligence in children with congenital toxoplasmosis, psychoses, dementia and epilepsy, culminating in an increased risk for suicide** (17, 22, 29, 81, 91).

Even though all these severe disturbances of mental resilience, concentration ability, behavioural changes and psychic disorders because of toxoplasmosis have been proven, magnetic resonance images (MRI) of the brain may show no abnormalities, even in the case of a Toxoplasma-induced inflammation of the brain. In 2015 there was a report about a patient with such an inflammation of the brain; an MRI of his head showed no anomalies (5). An MRI is not 100% reliable.

It is alarming that most of these severe health risks are caused in connection with a positive Toxoplasma IgG assay alone, and again the question arises if there can be a Toxoplasma activity that we can't detect with our standard lab procedures.

One of the most complete overviews about the symptoms of "latent" toxoplasmosis has been published by Flegr and Escudero (30) and by Flegr et al. (31). The impact on our health is much stronger than previously assumed, and the list of symptoms is long and detailed. The authors consequently describe high infestation with Toxoplasma gondii as a huge and underrated problem for the health of the entire population, a global risk. I do entirely agree with this view.

Toxoplasma can most probably reach and severely debilitate all organ systems and thus it causes such varied symptoms. The impact of Toxoplasma infections on our health is strongly underestimated. The reason for this might be that, due to negative laboratory findings, the resulting illnesses are not attributed to a Toxoplasma infection, or that the individual symptoms are examined only separately in single medical disciplines and thus the clinical picture is seldom seen as a whole.

6.5.   Methods of detection

This chapter is a bit tricky, but it explains why this disease cannot be diagnosed by means of laboratory results alone, despite medical laboratories doing their work with utmost care.

It has to be stressed that a treatment is not immediately necessary in case of a positive Toxoplasma assay. Toxoplasma may persist inside our organism for a lifetime without us getting ill. A treatment is only necessary if a patient suffers from an active toxoplasmosis and exhibits clear symptoms. The repeatedly mentioned diagnostic problems result from Toxoplasma's camouflage. While transforming from tachyzoites to bradyzoites they dramatically change their surface structure (76, 77) and in doing so they deceive our laboratory technology.

Three detection methods that are currently used are presented here. A fourth method, the lymphocyte transformation test (LTT) is available, and to my personal experience it is reliable, but it is not commonly used. You'll find details of the LTT on pages 211 - 214.

1)   Microscopical examination of tissue samples

This is time-consuming and difficult, and therefore not suitable for a large number of examinations. Many patients would also be less than enthusiastic to have tissue samples being taken. The testing order has to be clearly focussed on the detection of Toxoplasma, since several staining techniques are available which are not equally suitable for the detection of Toxoplasma.

2) Detection of pathogenic agent's genetic material in the blood

This is done by means of a PCR test. It is considered the "gold standard" in the diagnosis of many diseases. In the case of toxoplasmosis it has been proven that PCR testing only shows a very limited reliability (22, 45, 52). This is probably caused by the fact that toxoplasma is only ever found in the blood for a very short time (46).

3) Antibody determination

As a response to infection, the organism produces antibodies specific to each pathogenic agent ("immunoglobulins"). These will in the following be abbreviated as "Ig". If specific Ig are determined, it is a clear sign that the organism has coped with the corresponding disease. There are several types of antibodies, but so far only tachyzoite specific antibodies, mostly IgM and IgG are examined. **IgM** are produced in the early stages of an infection and are therefore seen as a proof for an acute illness requiring treatment.

IgG are antibodies, whose production is started few days after the infection has begun, and can usually still be detected even several years after infection. They have the task of guaranteeing a long-lasting protection. Unfortunately, animal testing as early as 1966 showed that not all individuals produce Toxoplasma antibodies in a Toxoplasma infection (48), a finding that has been confirmed again and again over the years (24, 53). In some cases, several test systems (Sabin Feldmann test, Westernblot, modified agglutination test) failed to identify infection, even when used together.

This is in accordance with the finding that tachyzoite specific IgG anti-bodies in *initial infections* are only detected with a sensitivity of about 82% by a standard test (66), thus there is 18% room for mistakes. This may vary for other tests as well as the standard one.

A Toxoplasma infection cannot be ruled out safely if the tachyzoite specific IgG shows a negative result, and this has been proven for several methods. It is unknown how long detectable tachyzoite specific Ig persist after a primary infection has taken place, but there are hints that they slowly decrease over years (46) and they might not persist for a lifetime.

Research about the reliability of laboratory results in case of a reactivation of Toxoplasma is unknown to me. Research has focused on investigating this reliability only in primary infection and in acute toxoplasmosis but never in chronic courses of the disease.

The first laboratory test for tachyzoites was developed in 1948 (70). Unfortunately, nobody knew at that time that this test only detects tachyzoite specific Ig, as is the case in the other tests still used today. The ingenious change in surface structure during the transformation from tachyzoites to bradyzoites was not discovered before 1996 (77).

It is also alarming that the usual Toxoplasma tests used so far, have been developed about 40 years ago. Microorganisms, including Toxoplasma gondii change their surface structure over time. It is therefore conceivable that the accuracy of the tests has further decreased over years, as Professor Robert Yolken of John Hopkins Hospital in Baltimore points out (93).

His research team also found other evidence for the low sensitivity of conventional antibody tests (93). Apart from the usual antibody tests, the researchers also employed a detection method for Toxoplasma proteins that proved to be significantly more sensitive than the usually used antibody tests (see. pp. 209 / 210).

Unfortunately, a bradyzoite detection is even more difficult. It was only discovered in 1996 that the surface structure of tachyzoites differs fundamentally from that of bradyzoites (77). Therefore, bradyzoite-specific antibodies can probably not be detected by currently used tachyzoite-specific tests. Furthermore, bradyzoites only trigger a very weak antibody response of the immune system (77, 95), which is why it is exceedingly difficult to develop such tests. For years it has not been possible to routinely detect bradyzoite activity in the laboratory. This probably has strongly enforced the opinion that they were "harmless".

To date (2019), there is no routine testing for bradyzoite specific Ig available. We have to live with a high error rate concerning tachyzoite detection and we are still quite "blind" with regards to bradyzoites and their activity. The normal clinical procedure, which relies heavily on these tests, needs urgently to be questioned.

This problematic situation is also well known to doctors in case of other diseases. If no reliable tests are available, we have to diagnose the disease according to its symptoms, and this is also possible in case of an active toxoplasmosis. The procedure will be described in the next chapter.

6.6. Diagnosis of an active toxoplasmosis in the doctor's surgery

Many possible symptoms of an active toxoplasmosis have been revealed by research (see chapter 6.4. p. 49 - 51), but single symptoms might well be partially caused by other diseases. Therefore, diseases with similar symptoms have to be ruled out or confirmed by means of suitable diagnostic measures. This is a complex process which involves intensive consultations and thorough consideration. Especially with a clinical picture that is so difficult to grasp as chronic active toxoplasmosis, all possible directions have had to be considered. This will be explained in detail in chapter 7 (p.61 - 72).

The patients I finally diagnosed with an active toxoplasmosis suffered from a combination of symptoms including pronounced permanent fatigue, muscular pains with a partially reduced muscular performance or cramps and concentration disorders. Frequent accompanying symptoms were profuse sweating, listlessness and dyspnoea with increased heart rate after only light physical strain. The Toxoplasma IgG was increased for only 60% of patients and IgM antibodies was below the limit for all of these patients.   In most cases the symptoms showed a slow and steady increase in the course of months to years, but intermittent progressions were also described, in which low-symptomatic stages alternated with stages of intense symptoms.

Please consider at all times: not a single symptom, but only the combination of symptoms is typical for an active toxoplasmosis.   An extensive differential diagnosis (see chapter 7. p.61 - 72) is essential. At this point I want to state that in a strong majority of the cases the symptoms were significantly reduced, often to an asymptomatic stage, by toxoplasmosis therapies.

Especially in the beginning of these therapies, this was hard for me to grasp, too, but I could find numerous records that these very symptoms in toxoplasmosis patients had been observed and treated by other colleagues earlier (see chapter 6.4. p. 49 - 51). However, in 2014 I found nowhere an overview of the complete clinical picture as it is seen in the doctor's practice. The knowledge of individual symptoms is vital. Since reliability of our laboratory parameters is seriously compromised, a chronic active toxoplasmosis is mostly diagnosed according to the combination of these symptoms and by excluding other diseases.

In the following, the individual symptoms will be described and the frequencies of occurrence which result from my case studies will be mentioned. In detail, these are my findings:

Fatigue: all patients described an unusual, mostly permanent **fatigue**, which resulted in an increased need for sleep. Nevertheless, prolonged sleep did not result in normal alertness or performance. This symptom occurs very early in the progression of the disease, usually first of all.

Muscles: all patients reported about **muscular pains**, which mostly occurred both-sided, affected arm and leg muscles, and were felt in the same muscle groups for weeks and even years, and often intensified from year to year. Frequently, a muscular pain occurred during or after a slight physical strain, e.g. pain of the upper leg muscles when climbing stairs. Especially in longer or very intensive progressions of the disease, the **affected muscles were tender to pressure** and the **muscular performance was reduced.** Sometimes also more **frequent cramping** occurred. In some cases, the muscular pains occurred at the same time with fatigue. They are also seen as an early symptom.

Concentration disorders: **93% of the patients** talked about significant **concentration disorders** and **disturbances of the shortterm memory. Word-finding disorders** were also a frequent characteristic. Many patients had difficulties in concentrating on several tasks (impaired multi-tasking), often a numbed feeling was described and that thinking was less sharp (brain fog). These neurological symptoms mostly occurred weeks or months after the initial fatigue and muscular pains.

Profuse sweating: 78% of the patients reported about unusually intense bouts of **sweating**, which often occurred after only light physical exertion as well as in rest, **especially at night.** The stage at which this symptom occurs in the progression of the disease differs individually.

Dyspnoea: In 67% of the cases, a dyspnoea (shortness of breath, here often in combination with increased pulse, from even light physical strain) was reported, similar to a medium-grade heart insufficiency and in 2 cases even similar to a **severe heart insufficiency.** This resulted in extensive diagnostic measures (ECG, ultrasound scans, cardiac catheter examinations and more), which could not reveal the reason for the heart insufficiency.

Lethargy: Patients (63%) often talked about **lethargy.** They felt permanently exhausted and had literally to force themselves to get things done. This is also to be seen as an earlier symptom.

Irritability: In 59% of the cases, either patients or family members observed a significant tendency for an **increased irritability and lack**

of self-control, even though this change of character could not be explained by the patients themselves.

Vision Problems: 44% of the patients reported having a disturbingly **"washed-out"** or **"blurred"** vision at times, particularly in periods of longer concentration or when exhausted. Still, opthomological examinations yielded no results.

Depression: In 41% of the cases, a depressive mood persisted, which led to a **depression** that needed treatment in 2 of the cases. In these cases, the quality of life was seriously affected.

Sleep disorders: 38% suffered from nocturnal unrest and insomnia, which was independent of the sweating. This was expressed in pronounced sleep maintenance insomnia, and getting back to sleep after waking up at night was also very difficult for these patients.

Vertigo: 37% of the patients described an unfocused vertigo, at times including gait disturbances and a slightly impaired motor-coordination. In consultation they often reported about frequently "bumping" into tables, chairs or door frames.   They also noticed a decrease in fine coordinated movements, and they had become more "clumsy", and often they would let fall things involuntarily.

Anxiety: 33% of the patients were suffering from anxieties, which could not be attributed to a cause, but which improved significantly with treatment for toxoplasmosis. Patients literally didn't know why they were anxious. These anxieties often occur only years after the other symptoms have been described.

Oedema: 33% of the patients reported **soft tissue swelling and at times also slight water retention, particularly in the hands and feet,** which improved with therapy.   In two cases there had already been lipoedema, a combination of oedema and swollen fat tissue, diagnosed. In both cases this was reduced significantly with therapy.

Joint Pain: Patients also reported about **morning stiffness (30%), morning pains with first movement of joints ("run-in" pain),** that often lasted for up to 30 minutes, as well as **general joint pains.** I never observed obvious joint inflammation with swelling of the joints or burning sensations, as can be observed in rheumatic diseases. **My patients did not report about migrating joint pains, as are typical in borreliosis.**

Patients often talk about just one of these symptoms initially, and usually fatigue is mentioned first. Many people tend to judge this, along with the muscular pains, the concentration disorders, the lack of performance, profuse sweating and further symptoms to be age-related complaints or signs of wear with increasing age and thus they don't talk about them, even though they are definitely troubled by being unusually tired and constantly having muscular pains or concentration disorders at the age of 30 or 50.

The decisive indicators for an active toxoplasmosis are found only after detailed consultations according to the combination of symptoms. The doctor then has the difficult task of enquiring about all symptoms and also considering other possible causes. This leads us to the next chapter, the differential diagnosis.

7.   Differential diagnosis – the evaluation of disease etiology

Especially when laboratory findings are unreliable, as it is the case with chronic active toxoplasmosis, it is very important to take other possible causes of illness into consideration. These are illnesses with symptoms in part similar to those of an active toxoplasmosis or which can overlap, and which should thus be excluded prior to treatment, either by appropriate laboratory testing, other technical examinations or by thoroughly examining the patient's history.

This collection cannot comprise all possible diagnoses in detail. One could write a book on that subject alone. We will start with the "simple" differential diagnoses, the "basics". These can be safely diagnosed by laboratory testing and only then we will deal with the more difficult matters.

A vitamin D deficiency leads to a severe fatigue and may also cause soft tissue pain, bone pain, increased cramping, reduced muscular performance and in extreme cases even cause a heart insufficiency. In the long run, the risk for osteoporosis (insufficient bone density) and broken bones is increased. The immune system is weakened by vitamin D deficiency and possibly the risk for certain types of cancer is increased. Profuse sweating and concentration disorders are not attributable to this deficiency. The cause of a vitamin D deficiency is too little exposure of the skin to the sun, which is even true for a lot of children today, since they often spend too little time outside. Still, the argument prevails that only 15 minutes of sunlight meeting the skin of hands and face would be sufficient to stimulate the vitamin D synthesis in an appropriate manner. Let me assure you that for many people this is not nearly sufficient.

During the growth phase bones suffer from vitamin D deficiency most severely and they never achieve their full density! Permanent office work, a darker skin type or obesity are also major risk factors for a vitamin D deficiency, and the permanent wearing of traditional clothing which almost covers the entire skin is a sure "guarantee" for a severe vitamin D deficiency, if vitamin D supplements are not taken on a regular basis.

A vitamin D deficiency can be reliably detected in the blood and remedied quickly with the help of high-dosage vitamin D preparations. Symptoms then decrease within a matter of days. It is crucial that the prescribed dosage is high enough (20,000 IU per day, mostly for 1-2 months with the exception of pregnancy where the limit is 4.000 IU per day). The dosage for children is in consultation with the paediatrician.

The reason for this high dosage is that if we suffer from a vitamin D deficiency, and can detect this in blood samples, our vitamin "storage" in our fat tissue has been completely emptied as well. Our vitamin D level will only increase significantly and be stable over longer time when this "storage" is filled. To do so, you don't want token quantities, but high amounts. I never saw side effects of these high dosages, and this therapy is a tremendous help for those who suffer from a vitamin D deficiency.

Vitamin B12, folic acid and iron deficiency as well as hypothyroidism can cause fatigue and further symptoms and sometimes also changes in the blood count. Assessed in isolation, they cannot explain the combination of symptoms seen in an active toxoplasmosis, but can act to intensify symptoms. Thankfully they can be safely detected in laboratory testing, and they are well treatable.

EBV (Epstein-Barr Virus). This virus is the causative agent for mononucleosis (glandular fever). In English-speaking countries, the illness is also known as "kissing disease" because it is often passed on at a juvenile age by means of close physical contact human-to-human. From age 40 onwards, almost 100% of humans are infected. Typical symptoms are fatigue, exhaustion, fever and swelling of the lymph nodes. The illness normally heals within several weeks, but in some cases, it might develop to a ME/CFS (87). EBV particularly burdens the CD8 cells of our immune system, much the same as Toxoplasma gondii. **Beware:** blood counts have to be evaluated cautiously; the IgM rate, for example, may be negative for an initial infection, and it is mostly negative if the EBV is reactivated later (possibly after years). In case of doubt, further laboratory testing, such as a PCR test is necessary.

> *An EBV infection can possibly lead to an activation of a "dormant" toxoplasmosis (45), much the same as an activated toxoplasmosis might prolong or prevent the healing of an EBV infection. Since both illnesses burden the CD8 system, their combined effect hits our immune system nearly at the same spot, which is hard to cope with, even for an otherwise intact immune system (see case 19, p. 137). It has already been recommended to consider Toxoplasmosis in case of an EBV – like disease, if EBV can not be proven (45).*

CMV (cytomegalovirus). This virus, along with the Epstein-Barr virus, belongs to the family of Herpes viruses. The presence of CMV in a population is about 40-50%. The initial infection generally takes place with few or no signs of illness. Fever, swelling of the lymph nodes, headaches and aching limbs may occur, and involvement of the central nervous system, the eyes, the lungs and the liver have also been observed. In humans with a normal immune system, the illness heals within 1-2 weeks, but the viruses may still survive inside the patient for a lifetime. They can become active again in case of a weakened immune system and then may even cause a very dangerous progression of disease. It has been proven that the simultaneous presence of CMV and Toxoplasma can lead to a significant increased risk of developing schizophrenia (22). According to the Robert Koch Institute, diagnosis has to take into account that IgM antibodies can remain negative during a CMV reactivation so that the development of this illness can easily be overlooked if a CMV/PCR test is not arranged.

A combined weakening of the immune system due to Toxoplasma and CMV might have a very disadvantageous influence on the healing process, similar to the combination of an active toxoplasmosis and EBV, as CMV also burdens the CD8 cells.

TBE. The former, somewhat awkward name of spring-summer encephalitis has been changed to **t**ick-**b**orne **e**ncephalitis, which means an inflammation of the meninges and the brain itself. It is a viral disease transmitted by ticks, and should not be confused with borreliosis (Lyme's disease). In cases of a TBE neurological deficits ranging from discomfort up to comatose states are predominant. Muscle and joint pain similar to those found in a borreliosis or toxoplasmosis are not observed.

From here on, the laboratory results get unreliable, which means that in the following illnesses a thorough anamnesis (history) and an attentive physical examination are particularly important.

Borreliosis. This bacterial disease is transmitted by ticks and resembles an active toxoplasmosis. The main, and from my point of view the most reliable clinical difference is that during a borreliosis, severe joint problems are predominant and these seem to migrate from joint to joint. Muscle pain and, after a long progression, neurological deficits can occur. There are also laboratory values for the diagnosis of a borreliosis, but these bacteria are located inside the cells, much like Toxoplasma, and thus the laboratory results are not 100% reliable. In cases of active toxoplasmosis, I have never observed the "migrating" quality of the joint pains which is common in borreliosis.

> *Caution: Borreliosis may, similar to EBV and CMV, be combined with chronic active toxoplasmosis. This is a very dangerous combination that needs a great deal of attention. If both diseases are active, both have to be treated at the same time to be therapeutically successful (see case 16, p. 125)*

Babesiosis. Toxoplasma and Babesia belong to the same group of protozoa, and typically Babesia are transferred via a tick bite together with borreliosis as a "co-infection". They multiply in our red blood cells and in doing so they cause an illness that is comparable to malaria with intermittent phases of high fever. In severe cases also jaundice and dark brown urine accompany the symptoms, and multiple little blood-filled dots on the skin may appear. Fever as well as the last two symptoms are not typical symptoms of a chronic active toxoplasmosis.

To diagnose a babesiosis, a PCR (Polymerase Chain Reaction), or micro-copy of red blood cells can be used. In case of intermittent fever attacks combined with the other mentioned symptoms it is advisable to take babesiosis into account.

Chronic cases of babesiosis can take place, especially when the immune system is weakened or a splenectomy had been performed. A detailed discussion on borreliosis and all its possible co-infections as babesiosis can't be performed here, but surely these can also combine with chronic active toxoplasmosis and need to be treated accordingly.

Primary chronic polyarthritis. This is the scientific term for **rheumatism**, a very severe illness in which the human immune system itself triggers a chronic inflammatory processes and destruction of joints. There are a number of laboratory values, but "seronegative" progressions are frequent. In these cases, most laboratory values are negative, even though a rheumatoid inflammation of the joints takes place. In contrast to an active toxoplasmosis, joint problems are the focus here. Soft tissue pains may occur, but neurological deficiencies with discomfort are rarely observed. The administration of cortisone preparations result in a significant improvement within a few days, whereas cortisone preparations are ineffective in the case of an active toxoplasmosis.

Polymyalgia rheumatica. This is a rheumatic inflammation of the muscles that leads to chronic muscle pains and to muscular weakness. Numerous laboratory values are available, but are normally only measured in rheumatology clinics. Even these values might be negative despite clear signs of illness. Neurological deficiencies and joint problems are missing in this illness.

In contrast to chronic active toxoplasmosis the ESR as well as the CRP are significantly elevated in most cases.   A significant difference to toxoplasmosis is also that the symptoms of polymyalgia rheumatica improve significantly under administration of cortisone preparations within a few days.

> *Caution: an active toxoplasmosis can be followed by polymyalgia, which might still persist after the toxoplasmosis therapy has been completed and which then requires follow-up therapy (see pp 171).*

Chronic Fatigue Syndrome (CFS) is one of the most important differential diagnoses to chronic active toxoplasmosis. The term of this illness is somewhat misleading, since the clinical picture includes among the omnipresent fatigue and exhaustion especially muscle pain with at times pronounced weakness, concentration disorders, sweating and further symptoms that can intensify over the years, and which might render a normal life almost impossible.

In the English-speaking countries this illness, which strongly resembles a chronic active toxoplasmosis, is also called *myalgic encephalitis* **(ME)**, a term that describes the inflammation of the muscles and nervous system. Since it is not yet clear if **CFS** and **ME** are the same or two very similar illnesses, the two terms are often combined as **ME/CFS**.
It has been estimated that about 240,000 people in Germany and about 17 million people worldwide suffer from **ME/CFS**. This illness has been considered as largely untreatable, which is unbearable for all involved.

Despite all efforts is has not been possible to find *the one,* definitive cause of ME/CFS, but it is surely a mistake to rate it as purely psychosomatic, because significant alterations in the metabolism were found in ME/CFS patients (59). According to my experience, a significant increase of symptoms after physical or mental exertion, as is considered to be typical for ME/CFS, is less pronounced in cases of chronic active toxoplasmosis. See also **"Addition in 10/2019"**, page174.

If a toxoplasmosis treatment is undertaken in ME/CFS patients, it is important to use a very low dose in the beginning, to avoid a strong initial effect. For example, clindamycin 2 x 150mg might be prescribed, to be increased to 3 x 300 mg only if there are no strong side effects. It is also advisable, to use also a reduced dosis during the combination therapy, for example Pyrimethamine 25 mg (daraprim) only once a day. It is sensible to treat carefully with a reduced dosage for a longer time than to use a normal dosage, as these patients are often so seriously affected, that side effects can be unbearable.

It is striking that Toxoplasmosis has been already directly adressed as a possible cause for ME/CFS (45). It is possible that other diseases can also be involved, but I am sure that Toxoplasma has to be addressed as a major pathogen.

The symptoms of ME/CFS and chronic active toxoplasmosis are very similar and possibly some patients, who have been diagnosed with ME/CFS are suffering from a chronic active toxoplasmosis, which in these cases might either be the cause of illness itself or a severe additional factor.

Fibromyalgia. This term is less of a precise diagnosis but more of a collective term, which describes pronounced pains of the connective tissue and the muscles. They can get so intense that even a slightly firmer touch can be painful, which can also be the case in an active toxoplasmosis. The diagnose is difficult, especially since many other illnesses have to be ruled out and there are no laboratory values available which can identify fibromyalgia. Typically, in fibromyalgia, "tender points" are very sensitive to pressure and are thus a crucial part of diagnosing the illness. Neurological deficiencies are not part of fibromyalgia, and the administration of cortisone preparations is ineffective. In several of my patients, a fibromyalgia had been assumed as source of illness prior to diagnosing toxoplasmosis.

Somatoform pain disorder. This is a more recent term in medicine. If a person is exposed to very strong psychic stress, the brain is flooded with stress hormones and a shift of the pain threshold in the direction of higher sensitivity takes place. The triggering stress stimulus can have taken place long ago, perhaps during childhood. Weak pain stimuli are then perceived as much stronger. Pain is of a high intensity and it is not "imaginary". An unusual fatigue, dyspnea, concentration disorders, visual disturbances and profuse sweating are not part of the clinical picture, as opposed to that of active toxoplasmosis. The treatment is handled with specific pain medication, psychotherapy and possibly antidepressants.

Depression. This is a very serious illness, which is unfortunately claimed too often as cause of illness if patients are suffering from unclear symptoms. The problem then is not the illness, but the false diagnosis.

A depression is marked by permanent weighed-down moods, frequent negative thoughts and listlessness. Many patients also lose their joy in life. Sleeping disorders and concentration disorders can also occur. Even healthy people may sometimes be severely affected, but for those suffering from depression it is a permanent state. The psychic symptoms are in parts similar to those of a toxoplasmosis, but in an active toxoplasmosis, the physical symptoms such as muscular pains, dyspnoea, sweating and visual disturbances are distinctive, and depressive moods are often "merely" an additional symptom. Or in other words, if strikingly many physical symptoms are present in the case of depression, it should be taken in account that an additional undetected deficiency or an undetected physical illness, such as toxoplasmosis may play a role.

Coronary heart disease. The coronary vessels supply blood to the heart muscle. If they get narrow, dyspnoea and a tightness of the chest with exertion occur, often accompanied by radiating pain to the left arm. This is described as "angina pectoris", which can be translated simply as "tightness of the chest". A reduced physical tolerance and increased bouts of sweating especially in stressful situations can result. These symptoms can vary, too. Angina pectoris sometimes does not focus on the chest, but it shows in a feeling of pressure and pain in the lower jaw, upper abdomen or back, at chest height.

Electrocardiogram (ECG) results *might* still be relatively inconspicuous under resting conditions, but an exercise ECG can achieve a higher predictive value of about 70%. There is still room left for mistakes, and therefore one should consider referral to a cardiologist or admission to a cardiological unit for those patients who have still angina pectoris symptoms despite inconspicuous ECG and exercise ECG findings.

Bronchial asthma / COPD. I must ask the pulmonary specialists to excuse me for summarising both illnesses in one paragraph. In cases of bronchial asthma, a "cramping" of the small bronchi is the main reason, often with an allergic background. In cases of **C**hronic **O**bstructive **P**ulmonary **D**isease, a pathological change of the lung tissue with an increase in little-ventilated "dead spaces" and a decrease in the number of alveoli represents the illness. Both illnesses result in exertional dyspnoea and can occur at the same time. Pulmonary specialists are able to identify them clearly and to treat them accordingly. But here one also has to be aware at all times, since the symptoms of bronchial asthma and COPD can be very similar to those of angina pectoris.

Chronic gallbladder inflammation: This should be one of the rather "simple" diagnoses, but it has its catches. I will list it here because a chronic inflammation of the gallbladder can also result in unclear sweating, fatigue, decrease in performance and aggressive changes of behaviour. The pear – shaped gallbladder lies in the right upper abdomen shortly below the costal arch and serves as a temporary storage for the bile, which is produced by the liver.

During the initial stages of an inflammation, and these can drag on for months to years, it often causes complaints in the *middle* of the upper abdomen. That is often an unpleasant feeling of pressure and bloating after eating, but a reduction of performance, increased sweating and increased aggressive moods are frequently experienced. The German saying "you stir my stomach" could then hit the nail on the head, only the partner is quite innocent when it comes to causing this foul mood.

Only in later stages of the illness the pain "migrates" to the right upper abdomen, and the gallbladder is then already clearly sensitive to pressure. Ultrasound can be useful, but gallstones can be missing or, in the initial stage be invisible in an ultrasonic examination. If they are existent at all, they sometimes can only be found with the help of computerised tomography (CT), or via an MRI.

Laboratory values *can* still be inconspicuous at an early stage, but *if* first signs are found in the laboratory, they are mostly a slightly raised liver value (GGT) and/or a slightly raised ESR ("erythrocyte sedimentation rate"). A "simple" diagnose of chronic gallbladder inflammation can thus be quite difficult at times.

This is just a brief overview of illnesses that can appear to be similar to toxoplasmosis in some aspects and that might also combine with it, and which then lead to very challenging questions. Differential diagnosis is difficult and the doctor needs to listen carefully and to focus on details, and, apart from lots of consideration, a thorough physical examination is a prerequisite.

Personal remark:

Instrumental medicine and laboratory diagnostics are precious means, but one should not trust them implicitly, and in case of inconsistent findings it needs to be remembered that they can't deliver perfect results at all times.

A frequent mistake of today's medicine is surely, that in case of unclear technical results, a psychic problem is identified much too quickly as a reason for the illness. The severe consequence can be that other possible explanations might not be taken in account any more. A doctor therefore has to deal with these "psychosomatic" diagnoses very carefully and responsibly.

Patient and doctor have to be tolerating and persistent, and sometimes a diagnosis may have to be questioned. It can sometimes take weeks or months until the right diagnose can be elaborated, but in most cases this enables an effective therapy.

Patients sometimes investigate on their own, especially in case of chronic illnesses, and this can be useful and important. I always try to deal with these findings constructively, even if the resulting discussions may be exhausting at times. The scientific field of medicine is so broad, that nobody can have a complete overview of all disciplines and new developments. Furthermore, the patients know their body and their symptoms well, and they sometimes may even be right.

Many important aspects of human beings (gait, posture, facial expression, colour of skin, auscultation [listening with the stethoscope], palpation, possible sweating, psyche and much more) cannot be gathered by technology so far. But humans have a natural feeling for that, and it can be trained.

Medicine requires, apart from a comprehensive knowledge and experience, an extensive empathy and skilful listening, a thorough examination and careful consideration. In long progressions of a disease, a checklist can be useful at times. Intuition sometimes also plays a role at finding the diagnosis and all this will surely not be replaced by technical procedures in the foreseeable future.

8.   The "Checklist Toxoplasmosis"

To organize my diagnostic procedure, I prepared a checklist organizing common symptoms and allowing for a rating of their severity. It has proven to be very useful. In the beginning of my case documentations I started with the first four questions on the checklist, but it soon became obvious that there were a lot more symptoms of active toxoplasmosis which were relevant for the diagnosis as well as for the evaluation of the progress of treatment. The list was completed over time and in its present form it is a useful tool, even though not yet perfect.

Not the single symptom, but the combination of symptoms is decisive for the evaluation, which will be shown on the next pages. It is essential that a thorough exclusion of other possible diseases is performed prior to treatment.

Since presently an active toxoplasmosis can often not be diagnosed securely by using laboratory values alone, the patient himself ranks the intensity of each individual symptom on a scale from 0 - 10, prior to, during and post therapy. Naturally, these rankings are subjective only, but as a doctor one should be wary of not taking them seriously. In my experience, patients consider their answers carefully and deal with the scoring system responsibly.

It can be assumed, that "equally severe" pains or problems are perceived differently by people, but each individual will realise if the symptoms have improved significantly or not. Sceptics often claim a "placebo effect" as a possible source for improvement, but it is highly unlikely that healing of so many patients, who had in most cases been suffering from severe illnesses for years, could be achieved by a "suggestive" effect.

The "checklist toxoplasmosis" is the result of intensive research of former case studies and a trusting cooperation with my patients. The listed symptoms are obviously not exclusive to chronic active toxoplasmosis, but enable a risk assessment concerning an active toxoplasmosis by means of the symptom pattern. It is also very useful to document a decrease in severity during and after therapy . "0" is always used for free from symptom, up to about "5" for average symptom intensity, and "10" for a most severe symptom.

From some doctors' point of view, lab results dominate the diagnostic process, as they regard these as more trustworthy than the patients' comments. I don't agree with this opinion, and no one gets well just because his lab results are "inconspicuous".

Due to my experience, the vast majority of patients handle such a checklist with responsibility, and since with toxoplasmosis our laboratory values are compromised, we have to trust our patients. It is astounding that some doctors have so much trouble doing that, since we doctors expect the patient's trust in our work as a natural prerequisite.

Since the symptoms are so manifold, it is advisable to always work through the complete questionnaire while working on the diagnosis as well as during regular examinations of the healing process. This is necessary, since neither patient nor doctor might otherwise be able to correctly evaluate the progression of the therapy. In case of "good" and "bad" intervals, I ask the patients to name the symptom intensities on the "bad" days.

How to use the checklist:

The basis is a completed history and pre-examination to exclude other causes of illness. When out of the 6 first named symptoms (the main criteria) more than 3 are inconspicuous, an active toxoplasmosis is not likely.

A risk for an active toxoplasmosis can be assumed if intensities of at least "5" for Fatigue and for 3 of the next 5 listed symptoms (including "listlessness / exhaustion"),

or

if Fatigue and 2 of the next 5 symptoms (including "listlessness / exhaustion") and 2 of the remaining ones are rated positive. In most cases this means that the patient names an intensity level of at least "5".

All patients with an active toxoplasmosis reported an unusual tiredness, which means that the missing of that symptom largely rules out an active toxoplasmosis. In case of intervals with "good" and "bad" days, the positive effect of therapy in most cases sets in stronger and earlier. If the symptoms are without variation and/or longer lasting the healing process is usually slower, and therefore the characteristic "intervals yes/no" gives a hint which course it to be expected in the treatment.

The more criteria which apply, the higher the probability for an active toxoplasmosis. The frequency and significance of the symptoms listed on the checklist decreases from top to bottom. The checklist is avai-lable in german and english free of charge as PDF on www. fatigatio.de (see "Fachartikel", below the interview).

In cases with short disease durations and/or lower disease intensity often only some of the first 8 secondary symptoms such as "morning stiffness" and "joint pains" are seen.

The criterion **"exhaustion"** has been added to "listlessness" recently, as this is the severe and most important symptom in ME/CFS patients. The criterion **"visual disturbances"** has a high significance when opthomological causes have been excluded.

The symptom **"unsteady gait"** / **"impaired coordination"** is a newer addition as there was still a gap in the description of the clinical picture concerning this symptom-complex.

The last 4 symptoms didn't show often enough or showed too much variation to be used as criteria. Still, they present a connection to an active toxoplasmosis, as they improved remarkably under treatment.

A combination therapy should only be prescribed if the Toxoplasma LTT shows a definitely positive result or if the symptoms are clearly decreasing during the initial 7-10 days of clindamycin therapy. If a positive Toxoplasma IgM should occur, this would be a reason for therapy as well, however in case of *chronic* active toxoplasmosis, the IgM is extremely unreliable. Please also read chapter 10, which deals with risks and side effects of antibiotics therapy.

Acknowledgement: Since February, 2019 I use, aside from Toxoplasma IgM and IgG, a Toxoplasma LTT for those patients whose results using the Toxoplasma checklist toxoplasmosis are positive. The experience so far is that in diagnosing chronic active toxoplasmosis the LLT shows a remarkably better sensitivity than the Toxoplasma IgM (see pp. 212 -220)

Checklist Toxoplasmosis

Mr/Mrs. ....

Age: ....years	**Duration.......................**	**Intervals** yes / no
Toxoplasma	**Ig** ....IU/ml	**IgM**.................AU/ml
LTT:	Date:	Date:................................
Treatment:	....	....

Fatigue	0 1 2 3 4 5 6 7 8 9 10	0 1 2 3 4 5 6 7 8 9 10
Muscular pains	0 1 2 3 4 5 6 7 8 9 10	0 1 2 3 4 5 6 7 8 9 10
Concentration disorders	0 1 2 3 4 5 6 7 8 9 10	0 1 2 3 4 5 6 7 8 9 10
Sweating	0 1 2 3 4 5 6 7 8 9 10	0 1 2 3 4 5 6 7 8 9 10
Dispnoea	0 1 2 3 4 5 6 7 8 9 10	0 1 2 3 4 5 6 7 8 9 10
Listlessness Exhaustion	0 1 2 3 4 5 6 7 8 9 10	0 1 2 3 4 5 6 7 8 9 10
Irritability	0 1 2 3 4 5 6 7 8 9 10	0 1 2 3 4 5 6 7 8 9 10
Visual disturbance	0 1 2 3 4 5 6 7 8 9 10	0 1 2 3 4 5 6 7 8 9 10
Dizziness	0 1 2 3 4 5 6 7 8 9 10	0 1 2 3 4 5 6 7 8 9 10
Depressive moods	0 1 2 3 4 5 6 7 8 9 10	0 1 2 3 4 5 6 7 8 9 10
Anxieties	0 1 2 3 4 5 6 7 8 9 10	0 1 2 3 4 5 6 7 8 9 10
Morning stiffness	0 1 2 3 4 5 6 7 8 9 10	0 1 2 3 4 5 6 7 8 9 10
Oedema	0 1 2 3 4 5 6 7 8 9 10	0 1 2 3 4 5 6 7 8 9 10
Sleeping disorder	0 1 2 3 4 5 6 7 8 9 10	0 1 2 3 4 5 6 7 8 9 10
Insecure gait impaired coordination	0 1 2 3 4 5 6 7 8 9 10	0 1 2 3 4 5 6 7 8 9 10
Pressure in the upper abdomen	0 1 2 3 4 5 6 7 8 9 10	0 1 2 3 4 5 6 7 8 9 10
Headaches	0 1 2 3 4 5 6 7 8 9 10	0 1 2 3 4 5 6 7 8 9 10
Joint aches	0 1 2 3 4 5 6 7 8 9 10	0 1 2 3 4 5 6 7 8 9 10
Swelling of lymph nodes	0 1 2 3 4 5 6 7 8 9 10	0 1 2 3 4 5 6 7 8 9 10

8.1   Confirmation of diagnosis

After other illnesses and deficiencies have been excluded and the result of the "checklist Toxoplasma" clearly indicates an active toxoplasmosis, a treatment can be prescribed. The patient is to be fully informed that a 100% secure diagnostic confirmation before the start of therapy is sometimes not possible in cases of chronic active toxoplasmosis.   It is surely preferable to start a therapy only if an illness has been doubtlessly proven, but the standard laboratory values available today are simply too unreliable. They also allow no secure exclusion of chronic active toxoplasmosis   On the other hand, the illness is too severe and to simply postpone a treatment.

Initially, a 7 - 10-day trial therapy with clindamycin 3 x 300mg to 2 x 600mg daily is started, since this medication is effective against toxoplasma without being combined with other medication (9). In cases of allergy, Rovamycine 1,500,000 I.U. 3 x 2 daily is an alternative to clindamycin. If the symptoms decrease significantly during therapy, toxoplasmosis can be safely assumed as the cause of the illness, which then results in a subsequent combination therapy for the duration of 3–6 weeks.   If the LTT shows a positive result, a combination therapy might be prescribed from the beginning on.

The combination therapies showed good to very good results in all cases in which the initial therapy with clindamycin was successful. In cases where clindamycin therapy is not effective it is mostly not sensible to prescribe a combination therapy (see my original paper on page 15).   In these cases, the differential diagnosis needs to be to reconsidered very carefully.

The decisive medication of each of the presented combination therapies presented here, which work a lot more effectively than clindamycin alone, is Pyrimethamine (sold as "Daraprim"). It deprives parasites of folic acid and thus weakens them. Apart from its effectiveness against toxoplasma gondii, it is also effective against malaria and pneumocystis carinii (a pathogen triggering pneumonia), as well as cystoisosporiasis (a diarrhoeal disease) and babesia (a malaria - like tick borne diseases, see p. 64). These illnesses differ significantly from chronic toxoplasmosis and cause different symptoms.

Since the beginning of 2019 I work with the Toxoplasma LTT, which allows in many cases a confirmation of a chronic active toxoplasmosis before the beginning of the therapy, and this is obviously to be preferred. Unfortunately, there are a some patients who suffer from chronic active toxoplasmosis for whom the LTT shows a negative result. New methods and thorough clinical studies are urgently needed, but still medicine doesn't rate bradyzoites and their activity as serious threat to our health. For new diagnostic methods see p 208, and for details about the LTT testing see pp. 211 – 213.

8.2. Therapeutic objective

The first obvious idea is to kill the parasite with the help of medication, in order to heal the patient permanently. But as often happens, reality is far more complex. As far as is known, no therapy is able to kill Toxoplasma completely, and the human immune system cannot do so either. Why are the described therapies effective then?

It has been mentioned on page 38, that bradyzoites and tachyzoites live together in bradyzoite cysts (6). Under pressure of a healthy immune system, there are generally only few tachyzoites, and their and the bradyzoites' activity is strongly suppressed.

In a patient suffering from chronic active toxoplasmosis, the immune system, especially the CD-8-T helper cells, has been exhausted or weakened considerably, and thus the Toxoplasma activity can increase significantly. The bradyzoites are then able to crank up their metabolism and more and more of them transform to tachyzoites (6). In doing so, they cause increasing symptoms. But despite all this activity, as long as the cysts and their host cells don't set free tachyzoites, the standard antibody assays will render negative results. Significant symptoms can also be caused by bradyzoites alone (42) without the help of tachyzoites, and as has been mentioned, the standard assays are not designed to reveal bradyzoite activity. If the initial infection took place some 20 or 30 years ago, even the toxoplasma IgG may be negative.

In some patients the duration of illness is very long. I found one patient who had been ill for 50 years (case 5). This shows that it can be very difficult for some patients' immune systems to regain control of the Toxoplasma without the help of a specific therapy once they have exhausted the immune system and increased their activity.

If the pressure on the Toxoplasma is increased by applying the appropriate medication, the immune system gets the chance to regain control. Bradyzoites then cease their reproduction or at least reduce it tremendously. Additionally, re-transformation from tachyzoites to bradyzoites (26) can aid in the reduction of symptoms. We can assume that the tachyzoites "flee" into this shape to slow down their metabolism, and this probably enables them to survive the therapy, at the price of a significantly reduced activity.

From the point of view of a host, and this is us, this configuration is better for our health, and after the therapy the balance between the parasite and our immune system should be stable to our favour.

To achieve a long-lasting therapeutic result, it is necessary that the immune system including the CD-8-T-helper cells can recuperate and that the patient recovers completely. It can be assumed that this needs time, and so the therapy has to be carried out long enough. Therefore, a prophylaxis with a reduced medication after the actual treatment for the duration of several weeks has been proven to be effective and indispensable. This will be dealt with on page 204. After that, the immune system should be able to keep up an adequately high pressure on the parasites for a long time, so that disease symptoms will not be felt any more. Then the therapeutic objective has been met.

Acknowledgement: I am confident, that a clinical study would find proof for the thesis that the immune system including the CD-8 cells recuperate after an adequate therapy, but this will take time.

9.   Antibiotics – benefits, risks and nonsense

The treatment of toxoplasmosis requires antibiotics, which I undoubtedly see in a critical way and this is why I will express my position here, before entering into the description of toxoplasmosis therapy.

9.1.   Benefits of antibiotics

Today, lots of illnesses which have cost thousands of human lives in the past can be treated. We don't experience cases such as plague, which can be treated with antibiotics if identified at an early stage in our culture any more, and nobody should die at the age of 45 because of an untreatable case of pneumonia. This easily leads to the wrong assumption that antibiotics are not really important and that we should largely do without them.

The counterargument is that a comprehensive suspension of antibiotics in Germany alone would eventually cause a 5-6 figure number of avoidable deaths within one year. Why and how do we profit from antibiotics?

Antibiotics are designed to attack microorganisms, so that their growth is slowed down heavily and they are killed eventually. If pathogen bacteria reproduce in great numbers, such a therapy can simply be life saving for the patient and antibiotics surely have a significant meaning for the lifespan that is achievable today.

In principle, nature serves as a model here. Well-known penicillin was originally produced by *penicillium notatum*, a fungus, to assert itself against competitors. It breaks the cell walls of certain bacteria. Several variations such as amoxicillin have been developed from penicillin that has a "broader" spectrum of effects. This has the advantage that several bacterial species can be "busted" at the same time.

The therapy is less selective but the result is still a better chance of recovery. First of all, this provides for a good therapeutic success and so tuberculosis, pneumonia, pyelitis (inflammation of kidney pelvis), infected severe wounds, and even bone infections and much more have become treatable.

Previous generations of doctors sometimes had to sit and wait to find out if the patient's immune system kept him alive, or if it simply did't. Help was not possible for many diseases. These benefits of antibiotics should be kept in mind before focussing on their risks.

9.2.   Risks of antibiotics

One of the risks results from bacteria's ability to adapt to antibiotics and to develop resistances. Normally it is impossible to kill 100% of bacteria. Some survive therapy, perhaps by disintegrating the antibiotic, as is the case with resistance to penicillin. These more resistant bacteria get "selected". They possibly need weeks to recover from therapy, but their offspring will have a survival benefit and will react less sensitively to the antibiotic in the next stage of the disease.

In the course of years, an excessive use of antibiotics can lead to a development of germs that are resistant to several antibiotics at the same time. These "multi-resistant germs", such as MRSA, can only be treated with utmost difficulty. The accumulation of resistances to antibiotics and the decreasing efficacy of reserve antibiotics are a global problem that can only be addressed briefly here; this will surely demand an increased attention of doctors, hospitals and officials for many years to come.

According to data of the national reference centre at the Charité Berlin, about 6000 patients died in Germany in 2015 due to multi-resistant germs. This very grave problem clearly is the consequence of a too frequent use of antibiotics in medicine and industrial farming, but it can be reduced significantly through determined measures.

The infection rate with MRSA germs in German hospitals still was 10-25% in 2011. Baden-Württemberg (a country in germany) succeeded in decreasing that infection rate from about 20% in 2010 to about 5% in 2015 (Kompetenz-Center für stationäre Qualitätssicherung in Baden-Württemberg). It surely contributed to this success that general practitioners and paediatricians prescribed fewer antibiotics during that time (Veröffentlichung des Zentralinstituts für Kassenärztliche Versorgung 10/2014), and that the screening for MRSA prior to hospital treatment had been increased significantly from 1% to about 20%. But there is still a lot that's left to be done to achieve the high standards of the Netherlands, Iceland and the Scandinavian Countries, where the MRSA infection rates are below 1%!

Further disadvantages of antibiotics are that they may cause discomfort and nausea, and in extreme cases cause direct damage to the liver and kidney function, or even to blood formation. Apart from these unpleasant to potentially dangerous side effects, indirect side effects through the killing of useful bacteria may also occur. The complete ecosystem of microorganisms living inside our body, the microbiome, can get disturbed severely because a lot of "good" bacteria are under pressure and a some of them are also killed by antibiotics.

By using antibiotics, we are thus causing collateral damage. A well-known and very unpleasant side-effect is the occurrence of fungal infections of the mouth or genitals as a result of antibiotic therapy, for example with amoxicillin. As a side-effect after the massive killing of bacteria, space is made in mucous membranes, and fungi can make use of this. Mostly this is a fungus called *"candida albicans"*.
This fungus is periodically found on our mucous membranes to a certain degree, and can profit from antibiotic therapy, since its direct competitors are harmed with the killing of certain bacteria.

As a consequence, the overflowing reproduction of that fungus has then to be treated as well. This is a situation which we would prefer not to have caused.

It is a lucky coincidence, to which medicine has contributed nothing at all, that the microbiome is self-healing most of the time and that it is very forgiving. This is the only reason why there aren't many more side-effects of antibiotics. Thus, diarrhoea due to antibiotic treatments mostly disappear after we discontinue the drug. The ecosystem of our microorganisms recovers its former equilibrium without any help. If this is fails to happen, the microbiome of the gut has to be analyzed thoroughly and the disturbed equilibrium has to be readjusted. Preparations including living lacto and bifidus bacteria are used for that purpose.

> Such a rehabilitation of the natural symbiosis with our microorganisms should actually be a standard procedure, but this is sadly not yet the case.

The aim is therefore to establish a cautious, responsible interaction with this group of drugs. Using them "too little" would be dangerous, using them "too much" would mean we pay a high price. A change of views is also necessary with regards to the duration of therapy. According to newer findings, a long therapy of 7-10 days does not only achieve the therapeutic effect but also results in an increased risk for the development of antibiotic resistances (Deutsches Ärzteblatt 11/2017). Consequently, the old rule that a package of antibiotics should always be used completely to prevent resistances was discarded by the WHO in 2017.

Instead of antibiotics, I like to use a mustard seed oil preparation or capsules with essential oils for slighter infections and also nasal drops containing silver in my practice. But there are not always suitable natural remedies for all illnesses, so that the use of antibiotics for severe illnesses is justified. The patient should be informed clearly about possible side-effects prior to treatment and it is sensible to monitor the tolerability and effectiveness of the medication. In connection with the use of antibiotics for "everyday" illnesses in my practice, I keep to the following rule of thumb:

One case of antibiotic use per year, e.g. for the treatment of a severe purulent bronchitis, a severe purulent sinusitis or something similar is not desirable, but acceptable if natural remedies are not effective enough in the particular case.

Two cases of antibiotic use per year makes me sceptical. The immune system should really not need help that often. It's worthwhile reconsidering if there are burdening factors which could explain the situation.

Three cases of antibiotic use per year means that the situation must be handled with utmost care. There is a high probability for burdening factors that prevent a better performance of the immune system. At that point a doctor has to become vigilant and has to invest time in extensive consultation and thorough examination. There are many possible triggering factors. A vitamin D deficiency (see p. 50) impairs the immune system and should therefore be routinely ruled out in these cases.

It can safely be detected in a laboratory and can be treated well. A chronic sinusitis, chronically inflamed tooth roots, chronic gallbladder inflammation, chronic appendicitis, chronic active toxoplasmosis or in really dangerous cases, malignant illness are further possible reasons. However, these illnesses might not cause conspicuous laboratory values in some cases.

We can conclude that, apart from direct side-effects of antibiotics, there are clear indications that the risk for antibiotic resistance increases with duration and frequency of antibiotic use. Doctors increasingly prescribe antibiotics only for the shortest possible duration to reduce the risk for resistance and thus the burden for the "good" bacteria is also reduced. Doctors should make use of antibiotics as moderately as possible, and patients should not demand antibiotics hastily.

The treatment of chronic active toxoplasmosis nevertheless is different, since Toxoplasma are so much more resilient and persistent that we could not get a long-lasting withdrawal with a short therapy. Therefore, a sparing use of antibiotics in case of active toxoplasmosis is unfortunately not possible in most cases. In my experience, a shortening of the toxoplasmosis treatment is not advisable because it often leads to a quick recurrence of symptoms.

9.3.   Nonsense: antibiotics to treat influenzal infections

Especially in the first days of a cold, symptoms are caused to the most part by viruses. These are pathogens that are even much smaller than bacteria and that reproduce in human cells or in bacteria. They don't have their own metabolism, but have to use that of their host cells. Normal antibiotics, which disturb bacteria's metabolism, are ineffective at the beginning of an influenzal infection.

Antibiotics don't influence viruses at all. At that stage, physical rest and herbal medicine are a by far more reasonable choice (only in selected cases of a "genuine influenza" can it be justified to prescribe a medication that stops the reproduction of the virus). But if the viral infection persists for longer than about one week, bacteria start increasingly to step into the foreground of the illness. They use the opportunity to reproduce while the immune system is busy fighting the virus. A virus-induced cold then might develop into a bacterial sinusitis.

Even at that stage, the use of antibiotics is by not mandatory, but it has to be considered for each case individually. The rigidly structured world of work unfortunately has a negative influence here. If I offer patients different options of treatment for an infection, they often choose the shorter antibiotic variety out of fear of needing a longer sick leave. In doing so, they don't really follow my advice, but a general practitioner has to take those reasons into account.

10.   Cases with antibody detection

The following statements are based on my own observations and documentations about chronic active toxoplasmosis over about 4 years. The diagnoses and treatments were carried out in the course of my normal consultancy in the practice, so this is a case study rather than a clinical study. My decision to summarize the existing documentations about patients with an active toxoplasmosis in a scientific work only started to form in mid-2016, after I had been treating patients with that illness for about 1 ½ years. The medication I prescribed is approved for the therapy of toxoplasmosis. Doctors call this an indication-appropriate therapy.

This case collection was compiled independently and there has been no influence or contribution of third parties and especially not by pharmaceutical companies. The therapies are not cheap, but they are "good value for money" in the best sense of the word. More about this in chapter 17.

It was not the purpose of this work to deliver a final proof. This is not possible without rigorous clinical trials involving universities, possibly pharmaceutical companies and perhaps hundreds of patients. Rather, the objective was to document my experiences and to convince my colleagues of this treatment approach. As a single doctor, it is very difficult to perform a "full size" clinical study, so this case collection served also the purpose of arousing the interest of a medical faculty. You can read about the reactions of research and medicine in chapter 15.

In the original work, 27 treated cases are listed and analyzed – in the meantime many more have been added. Even if I consider every case to be important from the doctor's point of view, I will restrict myself to 16 cases here, which will represent a profile of the clinical picture.

The 11 cases from Group A of the case collection come from a group of patients who exhibited clear symptoms of an active toxoplasmosis and in which at least one toxoplasmosis antibody, the IgG, showed positive results. With a positive IgG detection, it is undisputable that these patients are carriers of Toxoplasma. But, the reliability of Toxoplasma IgG and IgM detection has only been investigated in primary infections, and they are only elevated in these *acute* courses of the disease.

But by no means does this prove that these values are reliable in a *chronic* course of an active toxoplasmosis. If this is caused predominantly by Bradyzoite activity, it is highly likely not to be detected by a Tachyzoite specific lab test – these are just not relevant in chronic courses of the disease. (see pp. 53/54). A negative Toxoplasma IgM then just indicates that tachyzoite activity doesn't blast the host cells.

Only few doctors know about this, so it is still generally assumed that if the tachyzoite specific antibodies are negative the patient can't suffer from an active toxoplasmosis, even if he shows pronounced toxplasmosis - typical symptoms. Therefore, a therapy would not be prescribed in these cases. Nevertheless, in my chronically ill patients the IgM was not significantly increased in any case. The patients responded to the toxoplasmosis treatment very well, in many cases as far as becoming free of symptoms.

The 5 cases taken from group B of the case compilation comprise a group of patients in which the Toxoplasma antibodies were completely negative, but who nevertheless showed symptoms of an chronic active toxoplasmosis (see pp.135 - 155).

The symptoms were almost identical for patients of both groups, but patients from group B responded even better to the toxoplasmosis treatment. An additional case that had been referred to me with the suspicion of an active toxoplasmosis by a colleague will be presented starting on page 205, as well as two recent cases with positive Toxoplasma LTT results treated in my practise (pp. 214 - 220). These three cases are not part of the original case study and the statistics.

For all patients with a suspected toxoplasmosis, tachyzoite antibodies were determined (IgG: positive from 8.8 IU/ml; IgM: positive from 10 AU/ml) and individual symptoms gathered by means of a questionnaire. "0" in this case means free from symptoms and "10", the upper end of the scale, the most intensive symptoms or pains.

A frequently used objection against that type of diagnosis is that the perception may be different from person to person. It is the combination of symptoms which is decisive and not the individual intensities, which are naturally perceived differently by each patient. In any case, a reduction of symptoms from 8 or 9 to 1 or 0 is a very good success, and at the moment there is no more precise method established to record the illness and to document the healing process of an chronic active toxoplasmosis.

Some sceptics explain the efficiency of toxoplasmosis therapies by saying that "Placebo effects" are the reasons of improvement. Please read the case studies and decide for yourself if it would be possible to treat so many severely affected patients that effectively by means of "placebo effects". After 25 years of professional experience I don't think that that would be possible.

Personal remark: The reasons for the treatment in the cases I describe were exclusively the patients' severe illnesses due to an active toxoplasmosis. All patients have been informed diligently about the medical background, as well as the effects and side-effects of the prescribed medication prior to treatment. Their illnesses showed significant similarities. Most patients had been ill for years and already had undergone many diagnostic and therapeutic processes.

The initial treatment with clindamycin had only been prescribed after other illnesses had been ruled out and when the combination of symptoms showed a high probability for an active toxoplasmosis. The assessment of that risk was carried out by using the "checklist toxoplasmosis" presented on p. 79. A combination therapy was prescribed if that initial therapy yielded a significant improvement after 7 but not longer than 10 days.

The documentations do not show only long and severe medical histories, but also a very good gain in health and quality of life for patients after the therapy. In the course of these treatments I became more and more convinced that in such cases one simply couldn't make the decision for a treatment dependent on hitherto available laboratory values alone. That is something I would rather not like to imagine with regards to the severe illnesses. At the present time (11/2019), all the named patients are healthy, including those who had to be treated because of a toxoplasmosis relapse.

Some of the case reports contain a lot of details, that is because the progressions of this disease often take many years, and this book is also intended for doctors. This also documents that the decision for a toxoplasmosis treatment was not a light hearted one in any case.

Case 1, Ms. Veronica M., age 35

In October of 2009, Ms M. was diagnosed with borreliosis (see p. 65) due to migrating joint pains and further symptoms and was treated accordingly. The treatment was difficult and extended about 6 weeks, but was eventually successful, the crucial factor being infusions with Ceftriaxone, 2.0g per day. Some weeks later, joint pains, morning stiffness of several joints for about 15 minutes and an increased fatigue set in. The migrating pains had ceased, so that a relapse of borreliosis as a source of illness was not likely.

In *January of 2010* a rheumatological examination was performed, with the resulting diagnose "fibromyalgia" (see also p 69). On *February 7, 2010* an appendectomy was performed due to chronic appendicitis. Afterwards, the condition of Ms M. somewhat improved, but she was still very tired and exhausted and did not feel healthy. In *October, 2010* extensive dental restorations were performed on Ms M. Her general condition still did not improve. Due to diffuse pronounced pains all over her body she still regularly needed a strong painkiller.

In *January of 2012* a general fatigue, lack of performance and a reduced heart and lung capacity including dyspnoea even with light exertion were documented. A vitamin D deficiency of 5.2 ng/ml (normal above 20) was balanced with Dekristol 20.000, still the general condition only improved very little. Slight water retention with tightness in the hands, feet and lower legs developed and at times visual disturbances with "blurry" sight occurred.

ECG and ultrasound examination of the heart showed normal findings and showed no explanation for the water retention. An inflammation of the heart muscle was excluded and in a stress ECG Ms M. was able to achieve a load of 125W.

The heart frequency during this stress test was significantly increased to 162 beats per minute. The heart had to beat at a higher frequency to achieve the necessary load and this meant a pumping deficiency. The reduced performance seemed strange to me in this case of a young, athletic woman, who regularly rides her bike. The blood pressure was increased to 162/80 mmHg during maximum load, but a moderate increase of blood pressure under strain is not pathological.

As well as these symptoms, frequent unclear evening sweating occurred since the beginning of 2014. In *June, 2015* Ms M. suffered from a severe *acne inversa* (hidradenitis suppurativa, a skin condition) of the groin. As a result, with a latency of about 3 months, there was a performance slump with listlessness, concentration disorders, muscular pains, fatigue and sweating. Starting in *March, 2016*, three surgeries had to be carried out on the abscesses of the groin, but an enhancement of the general condition did not occur.

In *April, 2016* laboratory values showed no abnormalities apart from a folic acid deficiency of 2.2ng/ml, down from 5.4. A substitution of folic acid for 3 months however did not enhance the clinical picture. In *June, 2016* the blood count showed a minor inflammatory irritation with a slightly enhanced CRP value, which did not explain her illness.

In April, 2016, tests showed Toxoplasma IgG 17.5 IU/ml, IgM negative. The symptoms had been persisting for 6 years at that time, for 10 months a definite performance slump had taken place.

The substitution of folic acid was stopped immediately since Toxo-plasma are unfortunately thrilled about a constant supply of folic acid, and we shouldn't make it too easy for them.

Therapy: after a one-week therapy with clindamycin 600mg 2x1 an improvement of most symptoms occurred. After 4 weeks of combi-nation therapy with pyrimethamine, calcium folinate and sulfadiazine, the patient felt significantly better. Since some symptoms still persisted, the therapy was prolonged for another 2 weeks. After 6 weeks of medication, the patient was almost free from symptoms. Fatigue and sweating continued to decrease after the end of therapy.

Comment: in the medical history there were several factors that burdened the otherwise healthy young woman's immune system: borreliosis, chronic appendicitis, dental status that needed restoration and finally severe purulent acne. The patient had been suffering from morning stiffness, muscle and joint pains for at least 6 years, and later from tiredness, listlessness, concentration disorders and dyspnoea with exertion. These were symptoms of an active toxoplasmosis, which had worsened considerably after the onset of the *acne inversa*.

After the toxoplasmosis treatment, the patient never suffered from *acne inversa* again. This indicates that the performance of the immune system has increased after the toxoplasmosis therapy. Mrs M suffered from no side-effects and stated she would repeat the therapy if necessary.

Ms. M.: results and improvement of symptoms in %

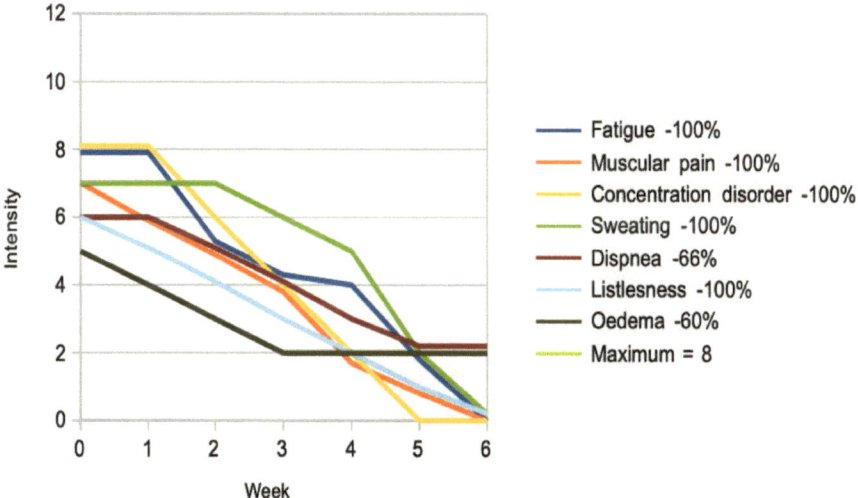

Time of the interviews: prior to therapy, after 1 week clindamycin, 4 weeks combination therapy and 6 weeks combination therapy

Addition 10/2019:

In 7/2019 Ms M. suffered from a relapse, the Toxoplasma IgG was rated 12,4 IU/ml, the IgM was negative, the Toxoplasma LTT showed, at 16,2 SI, a significant positive result (positive: above 3).

Considered, that the IgG has decreased in comparison to 2016, this indicates, that there has been no renewed activity of tachyzoites. So the disease and the positive LTT result can only be caused by bradyzoite-activity. During a toxoplasmosis-treatment of 4 weeks the symptoms vanished completely. Please see also to the addition on page 133.

Case 3, Mr. Udo M., age 60

Mr M. had a very strenuous profession and had been suffering from severe muscle pains and unclear fatigue for some years. He attributed this to his hard job, and in fact a significant spinal deterioration could be observed, which still did not explain the muscle pains or the fatigue. He was frequently very unbalanced as well, could not concentrate and had become very forgetful, which caused frequent unnecessary quarrelling.

An MRI of the brain yielded a normal result. A minor hypothyroidism due to a minor inflammation of the thyroid gland was diagnosed, but the condition of the patient was not enhanced after this problem had been solved. A vitamin D deficiency was supplemented with 20,000 units vitamin D per day, but this also did not yield any improvement. There had to be at least one more hitherto unknown health issue.

In August, 2016 the toxoplasmosis antibodies were determined, with **Toxoplasma IgG 26.7 IU/ml, IgM negative. At that time the symptoms had been persisting for about 5 years**, and after receiving appropriate information, Mr M. was prescribed clindamycin.

Therapy: initially clindamycin 600mg 2x1 was prescribed. Within the first week of treatment the intensity of the muscle pains was reduced by half, the tiredness improved significantly and Mr M. was significantly less irritable. Diarrhoea occurred, which improved quickly after stopping the clindamycin. Afterwards, a 4-week therapy with a combination of pyrimethamine, calcium folinate and sulfadiazine was carried out and a further significant improvement occurred. The irritability was reduced from 10 to 4.

Mr.Udo M. : results and improvement of symptoms in %

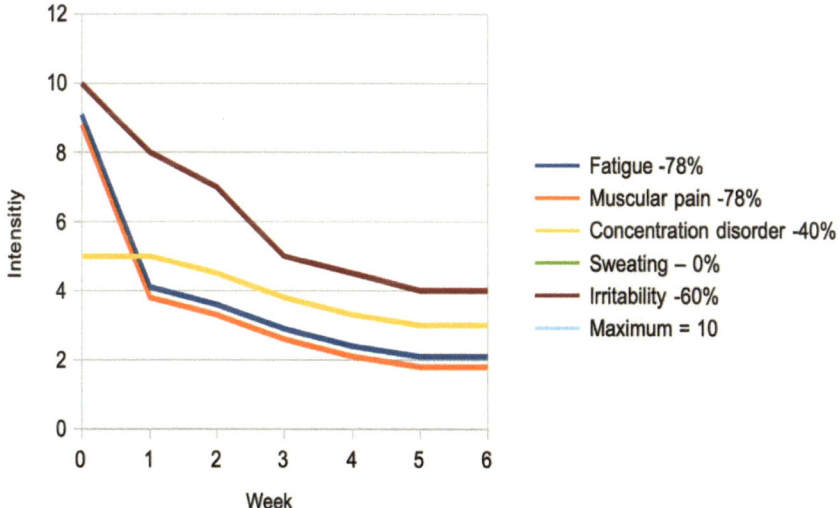

Time of the interviews: prior to therapy, after 1 week clindamycin, after 4 weeks combination therapy

Comment: By January, 2017 Mr M. had been almost symptom free for about 4 months. He had few side-effects and would repeat the treatment if necessary. It was remarkable in this case, that apart from the high efficiency of the therapy, the unbalanced temper and the frequently irritable behaviour of the patient had improved quickly and significantly, as was seen in several other cases. Even though the observed symptoms clearly indicated an active toxoplasmosis, Mr M. never suffered from sweating. This is no contradiction, since according to my observation that symptom is not observed in about 20% of cases of active toxoplasmosis.

Case 5, Ms Gerda M., age 67

This is the case with the longest disease history, about 50 years, and one of the most severe progressions. The result is a lengthy and difficult medical history that shows clearly how badly one can be affected by an active toxoplasmosis.

Ms M.G. reported that she had already been suffering from muscular pains and fatigue as a young woman. She had always had trouble straining herself and had always felt out of breath with even slight exertion. In 1995 she suffered from an inflammation of the heart muscle, the reasons of which could not be detected. Since then she had been affected by tachycardia. Also in 1995, rheumatism was diagnosed due to chronic joint pains, even though the rheumatism could not be proven in the laboratory, since she was "seronegative". For years, pronounced anxieties of unclear etiology had been persisting, which worsened with only the slightest trigger.

For at least 16 years chronic pains of the spine, the joints of hands and fingers, the hips and the knees had been persisting. An arthrosis was considered to be the reason for these ailments. Still this would have meant that a severe joint degeneration had been existing at age 51, which is not impossible, but unusual.

Since about 2001 a painful swelling of the hands and feet and morning stiffness for 3-4 hours, which is unusually long, were experienced. In 2003 an in-house treatment was carried out and here also, a "seronegative" rheumatism was diagnosed just as in 1995, but now in combination with a secondary tendomyopathy (severe pains of the tendons and muscles).

The left hip and the right knee were replaced by total endoprothesis (TEP), yet the joint pains hardly improved. Since 2006 a therapy with Lantarel, a basic medication for rheumatism was prescribed by the rheumatologist, but without the joint pains decreasing significantly.

Since February of 2010 an increased worsening of her general condition set in. Ms M.G. got more and more tired and weak and her pains got more severe. In March, 2010 Ms M. had to be admitted to hospital due to increasing joint pains, day-long persisting stiffness, back and abdominal pains, as well as nausea and an unusual tiredness. Colleagues suspected a flare-up of rheumatism and prescribed a cortisone preparation, which yielded only very little improvement. In light of the previously diagnosed rheumatism, this was strange, since in cases of rheumatism, cortisone should at least temporarily help quickly and significantly.

In 2010 Ms M. consulted me because of a severe infection that had been persisting for 4 weeks. I prescribed clindamycin 2x600mg and the infection improved significantly. To my astonishment, the patient consulted me again shortly afterwards and asked for a further prescription of clindamycin because it had helped her very well "in general". Since I did not have any explanation for that at that time and I always try to prevent an unnecessary prescription of antibiotics, I refused. An active toxoplasmosis as a reason for her numerous health problems was not yet "on my radar" at that time.

In March, 2013 an examination by a cardiologist was conducted because of unusual fatigue and dizziness.

Only a slight insufficiency of a heart valve with a very good cardiac ejection of 70-80%, a frequent diagnosis, was found. That diagnosis could definitely not be the cause for her problems. Furthermore, an intense dizziness and a pronounced insecurity of gait were found without any apparent reason.

Since the patient kept suffering from a continuing dyspnoea and an onset of water retention in the lower legs, a stress ECG was done in June, 2013. Due to the patient's pronounced weakness, this yielded only an output of up to 75 watts, which equals walking on level ground. I had expected an output of 100 to 125 watts. I could not explain the discrepancy between the good cardiological findings and inexplicably limited resilience of the patient.

In January of 2014 several laboratory values were determined by a specialized doctor because of severe joint pains. The rheumatoid factor, a further factor for the determination of certain rheumatoid illnesses (ANA) and several other laboratory values were inconspicuous and did not help any further. Since severe joint pains persisted, a cortisone preparation (30mg prednisolone daily) were prescribed, which only helped marginally.

In September, 2016 an examination was done by a phlebotomist, because of the pronounced swelling of the lower legs that had developed in the meantime. The diagnosis was a lipoedema (fat and water deposits under the skin) of the legs and a pronounced lymphatic drainage disorder, which means that lymphatic fluid could not be drained sufficiently.

By November, 2016 I had already treated several patients for active toxoplasmosis and in a renewed interview with the patient I realized that an active toxoplasmosis might possibly be the cause for many of her symptoms. Toxoplasma was **IgG 32.5 IU/ml, IgM negative. At that time, the clinical picture had been persisting for about 50 years and for 6 years the quality of life had been impaired severely.**

Therapy: Since the patient was suffering from pronounced pressure pain of the muscles, the initial dose was reduced to 3 x 300mg clindamycin as a precaution. During the first two days, the patient experienced increased muscular pains. Afterwards, her general condition improved continuously and after one week the overall resilience had improved a little. The patient also described her thoughts as clearer. Now combination therapy with clindamycin 300mg 3x1 as well as Daraprim 2x1 and calcium folinate 1x1 was prescribed and continued for 6 weeks.

Almost all symptoms improved continuously, the pain medication was reduced, the diuretic (Torasemid 10 mg/d) could be stopped due to a very good reduction of water retention from 7 to 0 and there was a significant improvement of dyspnoea. The ability to concentrate increased further, the listlessness and the muscular pains were reduced from 10 to 0.

As well, the previously very pronounced physical weakness improved and Ms M.G. was able to start a light physical training as the muscles were no longer sensitive to pressure. The bouts of sweating only improved slightly. Ms M.G. described that that symptom was very much dependent on the taking of a hormonal preparation that her gynaecologist had prescribed.

The therapy was discontinued with very good success after 6 weeks, but a relapse occurred after only 3 weeks of being symptom free. A renewed combination therapy yielded very good results after only 2 days.

By February, 2017 the patient used this therapy one day per month as a relapse prevention while being largely free from symptoms. Taking the very long disease duration of about 50 years into consideration, this will probably have to be continued for a longer time. She needs very little pain medication, and no medication specific to rheumatism.

Ms G.M.: results and improvement of symptoms in %

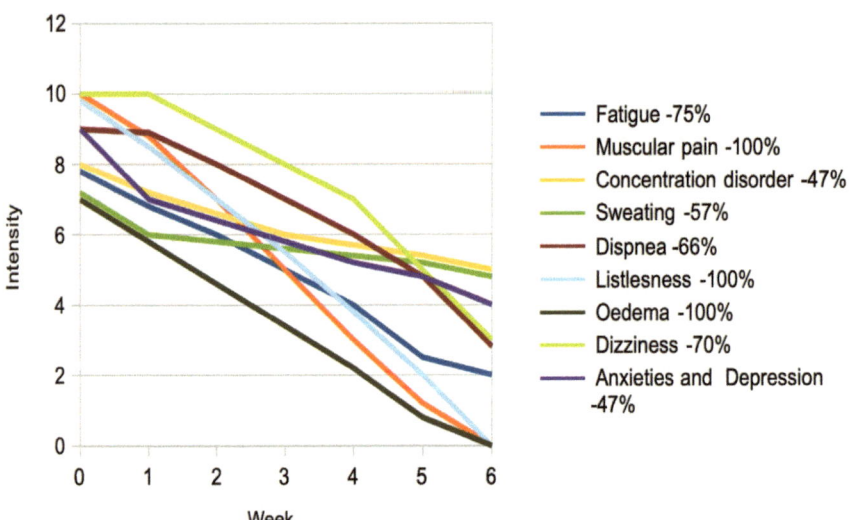

Time of the interviews: prior to therapy, after 10 days clindamycin 3 x 300mg, and after 6 weeks combination therapy

Comment: the improvement of symptoms and the enhancement of life quality cannot be put into words easily. Prior to therapy, the patient was so weak that she literally couldn't carry a litre of milk, let alone take care of her household. In the winter she could scarcely leave her home because her winter coat was too heavy. The permanent pains, fatigue, listlessness and concentration disorders made a normal life almost impossible.

The disease duration of almost 50 years is a very long one, which to me is the reason that this patient's symptom improvement does not come up to the improvement values of other patients. Even though this patient's symptoms were extremely pronounced, the level of toxoplasmosis IgG antibodies was moderate at 32.5 IU/ml, and the IgM was negative.

This case is most likely comparable to case 14 (p. 120), but in that case the IgG is increased more than threefold at 106 IU/ml. This comparison makes plain that the level of Toxoplasma-specific IgG antibodies yields no significance for the intensity of the disease.

Case 6, Mrs. Ina S., age 68

In 1995 a heart catheter examination was carried out due to a significant dyspnoea; a constriction of the coronary arteries was excluded then. In 1999 an in-patient examination was done because of frequent dizziness and a benign positional vertigo was diagnosed.

In September, 2010 a renewed echocardiography was carried out due to a continuing dyspnoea and yielded normal results, as did the exercise ECG. Still, capacity was reduced to 75 W. In May of 2013 a heart catheter examination was performed again, which still showed an inconspicuous result and the heart showed a normal pumping function.

In September, 2013 a part of the lower colon, the sigma, had to be surgically removed because of an inflammation. Two months after the surgery, scarring in that specific segment of the colon made dilation with a balloon necessary, and a polyp (a benign small growth of tissue) had to be removed from the colon.

Ms S. did not recover well from the surgeries and reported that she often felt extremely worn out, the muscles ached with even the slightest strain and she had significantly less energy. She could not get anything done in her household, felt listless, constantly tired and often had bouts of sweating. She had severe sleep disorders and had become very forgetful.

In June, 2016 a knee TEP (an artificial knee joint) was implanted, however the symptoms still increased afterwards and by now the upper leg muscles hurt with climbing stairs, and the dyspnoea and the concentration disorders increased even further.

In October, 2016 laboratory values showed blood count and CK (a muscle-related value) normal, CRP (inflammation value) slightly increased at 0.58, **Toxoplasma IgG 35.7 IU/ml, IgM negative. At that time the clinical picture had been persisting for about 38 months.**

Therapy: clindamycin 2 x 600mg was prescribed and the symptoms improved within one week under therapy. With good effect and tolerability, no combination therapy was initiated but clindamycin was prescribed for another three weeks. Despite extremely pronounced symptoms, the therapy could be carried out with only prescribing clindamycin 600mg 2x1 for a duration of one month. By January, 2017 Ms S.I. had been free from symptoms for 2 ½ months.

Mrs. Ina S.: results and improvement of symptoms in %

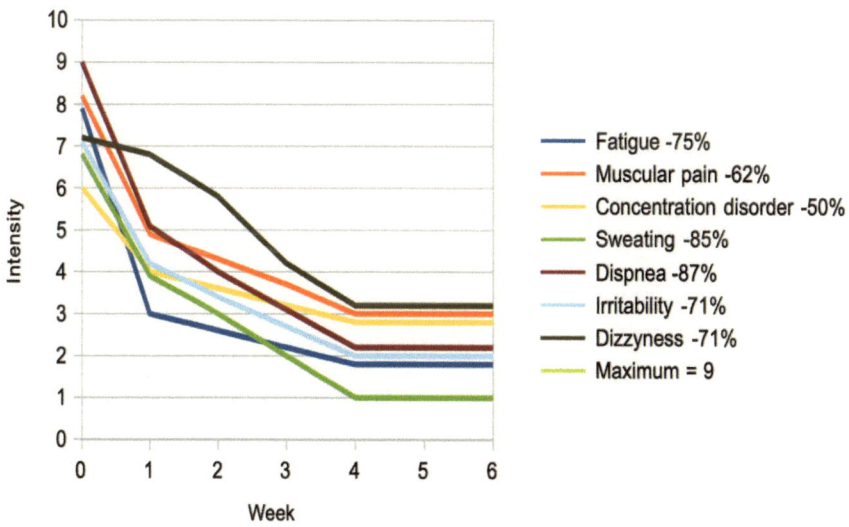

Fatigue -75%
Muscular pain -62%
Concentration disorder -50%
Sweating -85%
Dispnea -87%
Irritability -71%
Dizzyness -71%
Maximum = 9

Time of the interviews: prior to therapy, after one week of clindamycin 2 x 600mg, and after 4 weeks clindamycine 2 x 600mg

Comment: The symptoms started to be conspicuous after a colitis and a resulting surgery and significant worsening occurred after a second surgery (knee TEP).

The time frame seems to indicate that a pre-existing toxoplasmosis had changed to a more active state due to the patient´s weakening after the surgeries. The sleep disorders also improved from 7 to 2, which is a symptom reduction of 71%. Ms S.I. experienced no side effects and would repeat the therapy if necessary. Since the toxoplasmosis – treatment she never suffered from exertional dyspnoea again.

Case 8, Ms Charlotte S., age 63

Ms C.S. had been suffering from persistent muscular pains for a long time, when in 2003 a suspicion of a myopathy in terms of muscular pains was voiced in a neurological clinic. A physical examination and the examination of the muscles by means of electric stimuli yielded inconspicuous results. A biopsy (examination of a piece of tissue) of the muscle tissue was considered, but was ultimately not carried out.

In 2004, an examination by a cardiologist was done due to the unclear drop in performance, significant daytime fatigue and listlessness. The exercise ECG was progressing well up to 125 W (a medium level of strain), then a pronounced muscular fatigue and increase in blood pressure resulted in the termination of the ECG. A right-heart catheter showed only slightly increased pressure values in the heart with exertion. The long-term ECG yielded an inconspicuous result.

Due to severe running-in pains in multiple joints and strainindependent muscular and joint pains, a rheumatological examination was carried out in 2016. A basic therapy for rheumatism with methotrexate was considered, but initially not started.

In a consultation in October of 2016 the unclear muscular pains, fatigue and concentration disorders moved to the forefront. It became evident that the symptoms had been persisting for about 15 years, with an abnormal muscle soreness after only light physical exertion. Additionally, a dyspnoea with an intensity of 6 on the Toxoplasmosis Checklist along with physical exertion and swelling of the connective tissue in the hands and lower legs with a rated intensity of 8 was found.

The condition progressed in 3-4 month intervals with few symptoms, followed by an up to 10-day long aggravation with severe muscular pains, morning stiffness, listlessness, concentration disorders, fatigue and word-finding disorders, which was striking. Especially the word-finding disorders and the short-term memory impairment had been increasing significantly for the last 2-3 years.

In November of 2016 the muscle enzyme CK showed a slight increase at 212 IU/l, the **Toxoplasma IgG was increased at 38.4 IU/ml, the IgM was negative,** and **the disease had been persisting for about 15 years.** Since an extensive diagnostic had already been carried out before and many symptoms of an active toxoplasmosis were found, a therapy was initiated.

Therapy: clindamycin 600mg 2x1 was prescribed and consequently muscular pains and fatigue improved slightly from the third day onwards. After one week, the morning stiffness and muscular pains were gone, and the fatigue and concentration disorders had been reduced from 10 to 2. Listlessness had been halved from 10 to 5, and dizziness had been reduced from 5 to 3.

A combination therapy with Daraprim, calcium folinate and sulfadiazine helped to improve the symptomatic further, but the efficacy was reduced after about 14 days. Sulfadiazine was replaced by clindamycin 600mg 2x1, which led to a continuous improvement. Also, unexplained, intermittently unclear "blurry" sight disappeared completely. Despite a most intensive active toxoplasmosis no sweating was recorded.

Ms S.C.: results and improvement of symptoms in %

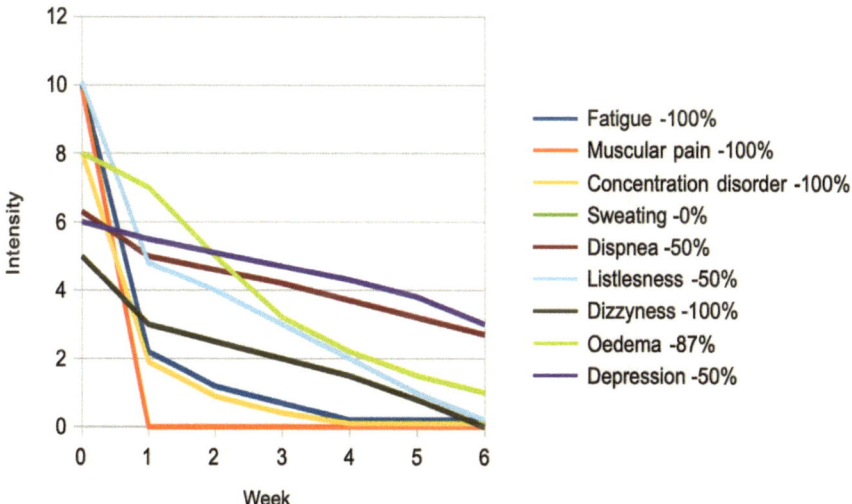

Time of the interviews: prior to therapy, after one week of clinda-mycin, and after 4 weeks of combination therapy

Comment: it was noticeable that the effect of the therapy set in very quickly. I have witnessed such a fast onset of therapy in other patients with intermittent progressions also (see the next case). Ms S. tolerated the therapy without side-effects and would repeat it if necessary. By the end of January, 2017 she was free from symptoms and she is still like that today.

The patient smokes, and a COPD persists. For safety reasons, a further exercise-ECG was carried out following the end of therapy in the beginning of 1/2017 and this was inconspicuous up to 100 W. Since the toxoplasmosis-treatment she never suffered from exertional dyspnoea again.

Case 11, Ms Maren K., age 39

Ms K. reported that she had been suffering from pronounced fatigue, sleeping disorders (rated 9) with profuse sweating at night (9), all-over muscle and joint pains (6) for at least nine years. She often felt cold and was constantly very tired and exhausted (10).

Since about 2012, diffuse abdominal pains and diarrhoea persisted (10), but apart from a minor gastritis, gastroscopy and colonoscopy yielded no significant results. The continuous fatigue was worsened by nocturnal restlessness, profuse sweating, and an unusual forgetfulness (rated 6) set in. Also, axillary swelling of the lymph nodes (7) as well as discrete oedema of hands and lower legs with feeling of pressure was observed.

Ms MK. also suffered from severe anxiety of unknown cause and depressive moods (9), as well as from a pronounced irritability and impatience (10), which occurred without significant reason. She explained that since the beginning of 2016 she felt cold in the evening even though her nocturnal sweating and further symptoms had worsened.

The entire disease activity revolved around intervals of 2-3 weeks, which means that 2-3 "good" weeks" were followed by several days in which she was very severely ill from all above mentioned symptoms, then all symptoms decreased slightly, until the next interval.

In March, 2016 a colonoscopy was repeated, which again yielded normal results. In June, 2016 dyspnoea with exertion and a pronounced cardiac unrest developed.

In October 2016 the laboratory values for blood count, muscle enzyme (CK) and an inflammation value (CRP) were normal, with an **increased Toxoplasma IgG at 68.5 IU/ml and IgM at 3.32 AU/ml. At that time the symptoms had been persisting for about 9 years.**

Therapy: Under 2 x 600mg clindamycin, the muscular pains increased within the first 4-5 days, and even palpable swelling of the muscles occurred, but at the same time dyspnoea and joint pains decreased. After 9 days altogether, the muscular swelling had disappeared.

Ms K.: results and improvement of symptoms in %

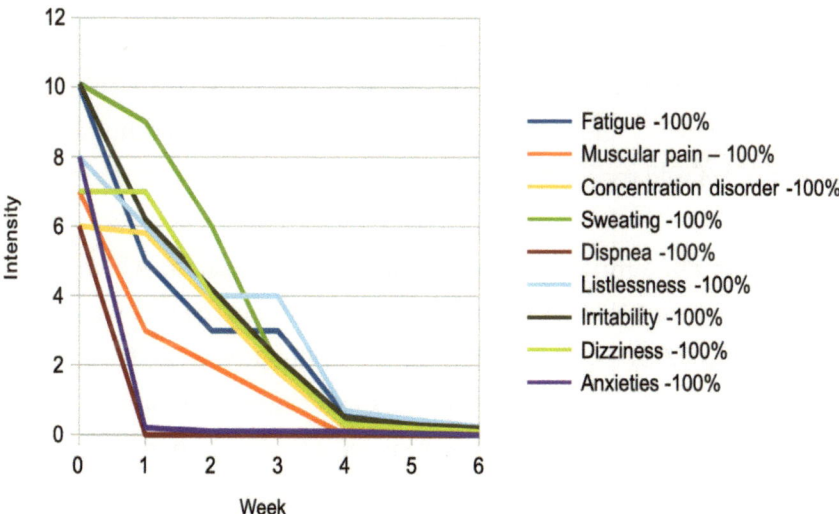

Time of the interviews: prior to therapy, after one week of clinda-mycine, and after 4 weeks of combination therapy

During her first week of therapy the patient experienced increased feelings of anxiety, which improved significantly after 9 days and a combination therapy with Daraprim, sulfadiazine and calcium folinate was prescribed. After 5 days of combination therapy the muscular pains and anxieties had been reduced to 0. Bowel symptoms also showed a complete remission as treatment progressed. Swelling of the lymph nodes no longer occurred, and water retention disappeared. In a concluding interview in January 2017, the patient had been free from symptoms for about 6 weeks.

Comment: Some patients report a slight increase in muscular symptoms within the first three days of initial clindamycin treatment. In this case, a palpable swelling of the muscles and an increase in anxiety occurred before a significant improvement set in. Therefore, I now prefer to reduce the initial clindamycin treatment to 3 x 300 mg in cases with equally intensive symptoms. Ms. K. suffered minor side effects and would repeat the treatment if necessary.

Significant abdominal symptoms due to Toxoplasma, which often result in gastroscopy or colonoscopy also occurred in the following case, as well as in cases 12, 21 and 20 (see the original paper). It has been known for a long time that Toxoplasma can cause an inflammation of the abdominal lymph nodes, resulting in abdominal symptoms (51). Also, an involvement of the stomach (34) and the liver (23) due to active toxoplasmosis is possible and could play a part in the development of abdominal symptoms.

As seen in case 8, an intermittent progression was seen here, and the effect set in early and explicitly also. All symptoms ceased completely.

Case 12, Ms Heide F., age 61

For at least 15 years, unclear muscular pains of the finger joints, both hips, the knees and the elbows, as well as morning stiffness had been persisting. A related clarification in a specialized clinic yielded no significant results. A vitamin D deficiency had been treated in 2011, but the numerous complaints were only slightly reduced afterwards.

Ms F. reported that she had been suffering from permanent fatigue, listlessness, a pronounced dyspnoea at even light physical strain (up to 10), and intensive bouts of sweating and frequent dizziness (up to 6) for about 10 years. All female members of her family had suffered from post-menopausal sweating, but her symptoms were most severe.

Her legs had been continuously tight and swollen (rated 10) for years. Furthermore, she had been suffering from severe concentration disorders, frequent blurry sight with intensities rated 8. She had been particularly irritable and impatient, and had been experiencing unclear anxieties and an unexplained tremor in the mornings.

In 2012, the temporary administration of a cortisone preparation (prednisolone) was described by a rheumatologist, and this led to a slight reduction of the joint symptoms. As a result, a basic therapy for rheumatism with sulfasalazine was prescribed, however this yielded almost no improvement and was quickly stopped due to side effects.

Ms F. also reported that she had been suffering for years from recurring abdominal symptoms of unclear origin, which were located around the navel and in the upper abdomen, and which were expressed in pressure of the abdomen and nausea and which she rated as an intensity of 7.

For some months she had also been suffering from an unexplained inflamed rash on the lower abdomen and the upper legs with an intensity of 8. In November 2016 I tested among several others the specific factors for rheumatism (AMA, dsDNA antibodies negative), of which only one, the ANA was slightly positive. The **Toxoplasma IgG was positive at 74 IU/ml, the IgM was negative. At that point the symptoms had been persisting for about 15 years.**

Therapy: clindamycin 2 x 600 mg was prescribed and the symptoms were slightly reduced within one week. After one month, Daraprim, calcium folinate and sulfadiazine were added. Symptomatic relief included reduction of visual disorders from 8 to 0, inflammatory skin disorders reduced from 10 to 2 and reduction of abdominal symptoms from 7 to 3.

Comment: At the end of January 2017, Ms F. was almost free from symptoms. She experienced "average" side effects and would repeat the therapy if necessary.

It was striking in this case that the pronounced swelling of the legs was reduced by about 80% under therapy. Similar changes have also been observed in eight other cases, but were most striking here. It is possible that Toxoplasma had caused an inflammation of the connective tissue, which then had resulted in water retention. The improvement in dyspnoea was also noticeable.

Ms. F.: results and improvement of symptoms in %

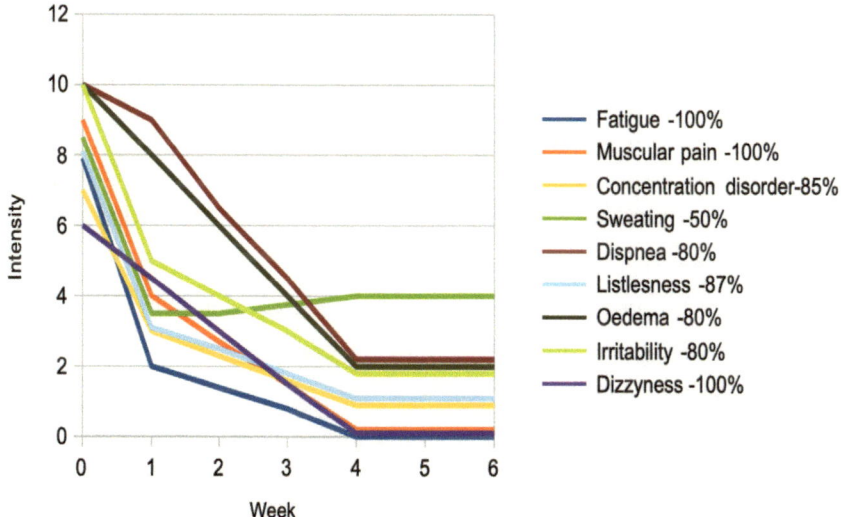

Time of the interviews: prior to therapy, after one week of clindamycin, and after 4 weeks of combination therapy

After therapy, Ms F. can cope with much more physical strain and can easily walk a distance of up to 6 km, which had been impossible before.

Case 14, Ms Anja H., age 47

Ms H. first came to my surgery in 2008. Since 1998, she had been experiencing pronounced pains of the muscles in her arms and back, and a fibromyalgia had been diagnosed in 2004. Several spine and knee surgeries had been performed. Ms H. was depressive, downcast and listless.

A gastroscopy and a colonoscopy performed in 2009 yielded normal findings, apart from a slight inflammation of the oesophagus. Due to the constant fatigue, sleep apnoea syndrome (cessation of breath during sleep) was considered, but could not be proved.

In June 2015, considerable recurring pains and pressure of the right upper abdomen (rated 10) as well as a noticeably lighter coloured stools occurred. The gall bladder had already been removed in 2012, but due to a suspected bacterial inflammation of the bile ducts, an antibiotic (Ciprofloxacin 500 mg 2 x 1) was prescribed. This led to a significant improvement, but this lasted only some weeks. About mid-2016 Ms H.'s general condition deteriorated significantly. She had diffuse muscular pains all over her body and a general weakness, and fatigue increased significantly.

On closer inspection it became apparent that the listlessness, unusual fatigue and muscular pains had been increasing in the last years, concentration and sleep disorders had been persisting for about 6-7 years and about 3 years ago, a pronounced dyspnoea (up to 10) had kicked in. Since 2016, the sight on her left eye had been significantly "blurry", yet the ophthalmological findings were inconspicuous.

September 2016 tests showed Toxoplasma IgG 97.9 IU/ml, IgM 3.06 AU/ml, and other laboratory values normal. **At that time the symptoms had been persisting for about 18 years.**

Therapy: in 2016 clindamycin 2 x 600 mg was prescribed. After 16 days of therapy significant improvements could be seen and Daraprim and calcium folinate were additionally prescribed. Since no sufficient improvement could be seen after 7 weeks of combination therapy, cotrimoxazole forte 2x1 instead of clindamycin was prescribed.

After another 20 days the therapy was ended with good results. In January, 2017 the symptoms had been improved for 2 months. She is at good health today.

Ms. H.: results and improvement of symptoms in %

Time of the interviews: prior to therapy, after 16 days of clindamycin 600 mg 2x1, after 7 weeks clindamycin combination therapy and after 10 weeks cotrimoxazole combination therapy.

Comment: the graphic had to be condensed with respect to time due to the retarded healing progress. The improvements from week 2 to week 10 occurred slower than indicated by the visual representation. The slow healing process can mostly be attributed to the long disease duration of about 18 years and the weak impact of the first combination therapy.

In addition to the changes shown in the graphic, further symptoms improved. The right-sided upper abdominal pains were reduced from 10 to 2 (similar to case 25), and significantly lighter-coloured stools no longer occurred. The sleep disorders and morning stiffness were reduced from 9 to 2.

Case 15, Ms Gisela H., age 59

Ms H's muscle and joint pains first occurred in 2010. An examination by a specialist yielded no rheumatological disease. About 2013, these pains as well as frequent herpes reactivation, signs of a weakened immune system, slowly increased. Pronounced fatigue as well as concentration disorders and listlessness led to significant vocational impairment.

In May, 2014 inconspicuous laboratory values for borreliosis antibodies, blood protein and vitamin D were recorded. CCP antibodies (which point towards a rheumatoid illness) were positive at 16 U/ml (normal up to 7). Light swelling of the hands and lower legs could be found. Ms H. was therefore examined again in a rheumatological clinic in July, 2014, but a rheumatological disease could not be confirmed.

In February of 2015 a laboratory examination was carried out. Borrelia antibodies were negative, **Toxoplasma IgG 99 IU/ml, IgM negative. At that time the symptoms had been persisting for about 6 years, and for 2 years the symptoms had increased significantly.**

Therapy: Initially, treatment was carried out with clindamycin 3 x 300mg for 20 days. The symptoms were gradually reduced. Afterwards, therapy was continued for another 20 days in combination with Daraprim, calcium folinate and sulfadiazine. The symptoms then improved almost completely. Concentration disorders had improved by 66% at the end of therapy, but continued to improve post-therapy (to "0"), which is why the reduction of this symptom is quoted as 100%.

Ms H.: results and improvement of symptoms in %.

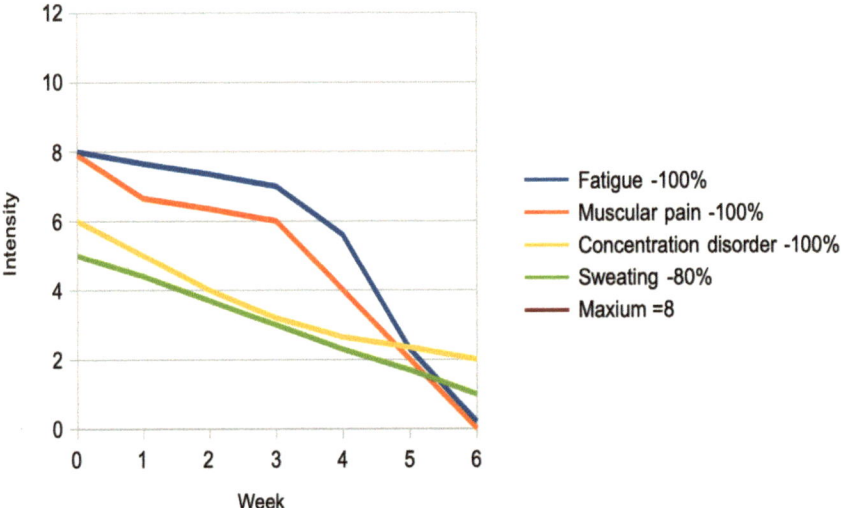

Time of the interviews: prior to therapy, after 3 weeks of clinda-mycine, and after 3 weeks of combination therapy

Comment: This is one of the first cases treated in spring 2015 and fewer symptoms have been noted, since at that time I knew only a limited number of symptoms of an active toxoplasmosis. The diagnostic schedule differs slightly. I decreased the clindamycin phase and increased the span of the combination therapy later.

Ms H. experienced slight nausea and a feeling of light headedness under combination therapy, which she rated as average side effects. At the same time, her symptoms improved significantly, so she wanted to carry on with the therapy. In January of 2017 she had been free from symptoms for 21 months. She would repeat the treatment if necessary.

Case 16, Ms Karin D., age 44

From age 13 (1985) on, chronic pains all over the body had been persisting. The patient had already been treated in hospital several times during childhood because of this. She explained that she had been examined for rheumatism several times, but the results were always negative. In 2002, sweating of unclear cause, a pronounced unclear fatigue and swallowing disorders were documented for the first time.

As it turned out later, there were recurring phases with pains in almost all joints, unusual physical weakness, tachycardia with exertion, as well as fatigue and muscular pains and the axillary lymph nodes were affected frequently from age 15 onwards. Ms D. has two healthy children aged 14 and 17.

In 2015 Ms D. had to undergo surgery of the lower abdomen. The progression after surgery was initially inconspicuous, but after about one month, a downturn with dyspnoea and a marked quickening of the pulse at even light exertion occurred. For reasons of safety, Ms D. was admitted to hospital to rule out endocarditis. A specialized ultrasound examination of the heart, TEE(transoesophageal echocardiography) as well as a pulmonary function test yielded inconspicuous results.

An exercise electrocardiogram showed a sufficient output of up to 100W, but this resulted in a noticeably strong increase of the heart rate up to 178 beats per minute. An increase like that might point towards a cardiac insufficiency. This reminded me of case 1 (p. 96). A blood culture was made once to rule out possible bacteria in the blood, but the laboratory values yielded no vital clues. Ms D. was advised so start psychotherapy and was then discharged from hospital.

Nevertheless, the patient's condition worsened within a few days and I re-admitted Ms D. after a telephone consultation to a different cardiological unit. Here the TEE also yielded normal results, but an exercise electrocardiogram could only be realized up to 75 W, which is alarmingly bad for a 44-year old patient. Ms D. now was also increasingly weakened and had very intense bouts of sweating.

The long-term EEG was inconspicuous. A moderate cardiac output deficiency NYHA II (NYHA is New York Heart Association) was diagnosed, still no cause for this deficiency was indicated and a depressive episode was suspected. The patient was discharged and came to my practice.

During consultation Ms D. was very pale and completely exhausted. Cold sweat and a slightly aggravated bronchial breathing were noticeable, pointing towards a light infection. The examination of the lower abdomen yielded no results. Blood values were normal, only the blood sedimentation, an unspecific inflammation marker, was increased at 38/58 mm. Only little information could be gathered from this.

Therapy: Due to the patient's threatening condition I assumed that bacteria were possibly spreading throughout her entire organism and that a sepsis was imminent. Therefore, I decided to administer infusions of 1 x Ceftriaxone 2.0g daily, a strong antibiotic. This is an unusual measure in a general practice, but it was inevitable because of the patient's condition. I was very relieved, when Ms D.'s condition improved significantly because of the daily infusions, and after 30 infusions only some minor symptoms remained. At that time the therapy could be ended.

About 4 months later, the resilience again gradually worsened, then intensive joint pains reoccurred.

In mid-November 2015, Ms D. explained that she has been experiencing migrant joint pains since youth; this initiated the suspicion of a chronic borreliosis as cause for the joint pains and a possible myocarditis (inflammation of the heartmuscle) because of borrelia. This would explain the efficiency of the antibiotic infusions, as Ceftriaxone is highly effective against borrelia. A rheumatoid value and the borreliosis antibodies were negative, yet I had treated patients before who had been suffering from borreliosis and whose antibodies had been negative. *Remark: It is known that active borreliosis often cannot securely be diagnosed by using antibody assays (see page 65).*
In February of 2016 the Ceftriaxone infusions, which proved to be very effective, were started again due to a renewed increase in symptoms. This time the 30 infusions of Ceftriaxone were followed up with preventive weekly infusions of Ceftriaxone.

In September of that year the patient revealed that she had been suffering from severe muscular pains, an unusual fatigue and a reduced physical resilience "as long as she can remember". She said she often had severe changes of eyesight and she felt very dizzy frequently. A magnetic resonance tomography of the head yielded no results. Ms D. also mentioned that she had grown up in a rural environment and that she had eaten fresh meat very frequently during childhood.

Toxoplasma antibodies IgG were significantly increased at 106 IU/ml, the IgM was negative. At that time the symptoms had been persisting for over 30 years.

Ceftriaxone infusions were stopped and clindamycin 2 x 600 mg was prescribed. As a result, joint pains started to increase rapidly after only a short time and the patient could not register any positive effect of the therapy. After some days the Ceftriaxone infusions were started again and at the same time, a combination therapy with Daraprim, calcium folinate and sulfadiazine was prescribed. Now a remission of all symptoms at the same time could be seen for the first time.

Ms D.: results and improvement of symptoms in %

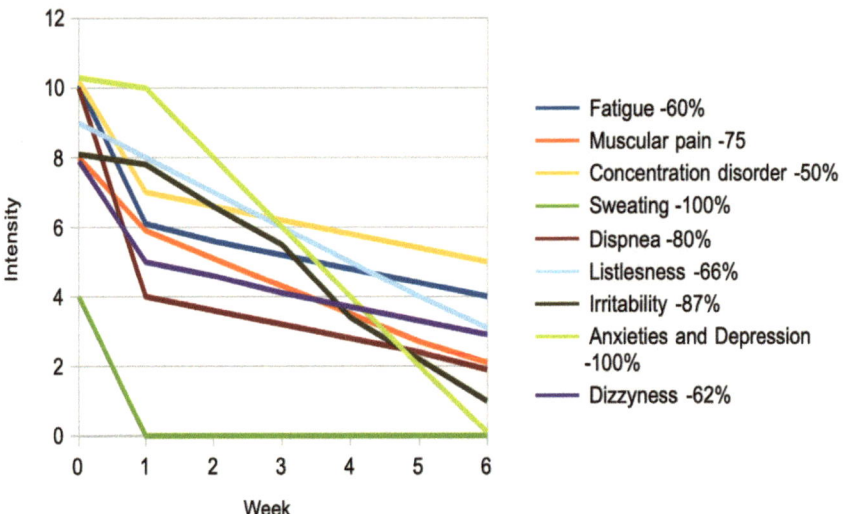

Time of the interviews: prior to combination therapy, after 1 week and after 6 weeks of combination therapy

After 6 weeks of combination therapy the following improvements in symptoms apart from those shown in the graphic had occurred: loss of hair from 10 to 1, sleep disorders from 8 to 3, slight swelling of hands and feet reduced from 4 to 2.

Comment: This is one of the most complex and difficult cases, and you can deduce that it has been a long and strenuous fight which demanded a great deal from the patient and me, since we had to handle two separate diseases, the symptoms of which were overlapping.

The pronounced travelling joint pains that had started when she was 13 years old and the later cardiac insufficiency had presumably been caused by borreliosis, and could thus be treated well with Ceftriaxone.

At the same time, active toxoplasmosis symptoms weakened the patient and that might have supported the quick relapse after the first Ceftriaxone therapy. The ineffectiveness of clindamycin can possibly be explained with the simultaneously stopped Ceftriaxone infusions.

Due to these unusual circumstances, I prescribed a toxoplasmosis combination therapy at once. Only the combined treatment of both diseases finally yielded an extensive improvement of almost all symptoms. As a relapse prevention against toxoplasmosis, a weekly treatment with Daraprim, calcium folinate and sulfadiazine was administered for another 2 months. After the combination therapy, travelling joint pains have not appeared again and today the patient is healthy.

Case 17, Ms Victoria S., age 37

The patient reported that she had suffered from several severe flu-like infections some weeks ago. Starting a month later, a pronounced swelling of the mandibular lymph nodes persisted. She said that she had never fully recovered from the infections, was very tired, suffered from concentration disorders and had pains of the shoulders, elbows and wrists.

Three months later her condition worsened even more. Now, severe muscle and joint pains all over the body, word-finding disorders, very severe bouts of sweating, hot flushes and swelling of the cervical lymph nodes were added. Dyspnoea and tachycardia now occurred with only slight exertion, Ms S. constantly felt very exhausted and frequently suffered from visual disorders, which she experienced as "blurry sight" even though the ophthalmological examination showed normal results. She was unusually irritable. Laboratory work showed blood count and ESR normal, other blood values including thyroid levels were also normal, the level of folic acid was slightly increased at 19 ng/ml. **Toxoplasma IgG above 400 IU/ml, IgM 4.75 AU/ml. At that time the symptoms had been persisting for about 7 months.**

Therapy: Clindamycin 2 x 600 mg was prescribed. After 10 days the symptoms had improved slightly, and a combination therapy with Daraprim, calcium folinate and sulfadiazine was prescribed for one month. During that time the complete clinical picture improved.

Listlessness initially rated at 9, irritability at 6 and visual disorders at 3 vanished completely. The word-finding disorders improved considerably, the tachycardia was reduced from 7 to 2 and the swelling of the lymph nodes was also considerably reduced.

Ms S.: results and improvement of symptoms in %

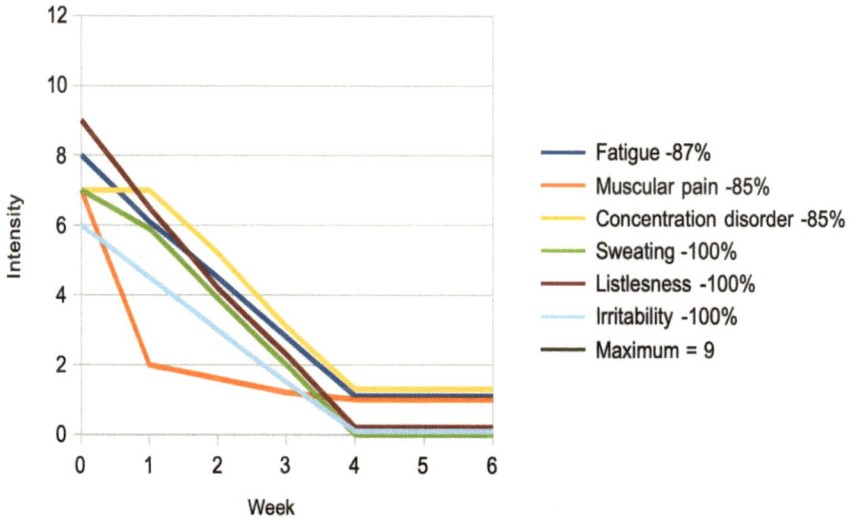

Time of the interviews: prior to therapy, after 10 days of clindamycine 600 2x1 and after 4 weeks of combination therapy

At the end of 2016, Ms S. had been free from symptoms for 6 weeks, but by the turn of the year she experienced a relapse, in which initially only fatigue (rated as 4), listlessness (5), muscular pains (3), as well as a minimal morning stiffness (1) occurred. A relapse after only 6 weeks is unusual, but the patient fortunately came to the surgery as soon as the toxoplasmosis symptoms reappeared. Renewed combination therapy was started at once, which led to a complete termination of the symptoms within one week. After 3 weeks the therapy was stopped.

Ms S.: Results and improvement of symptoms during relapse

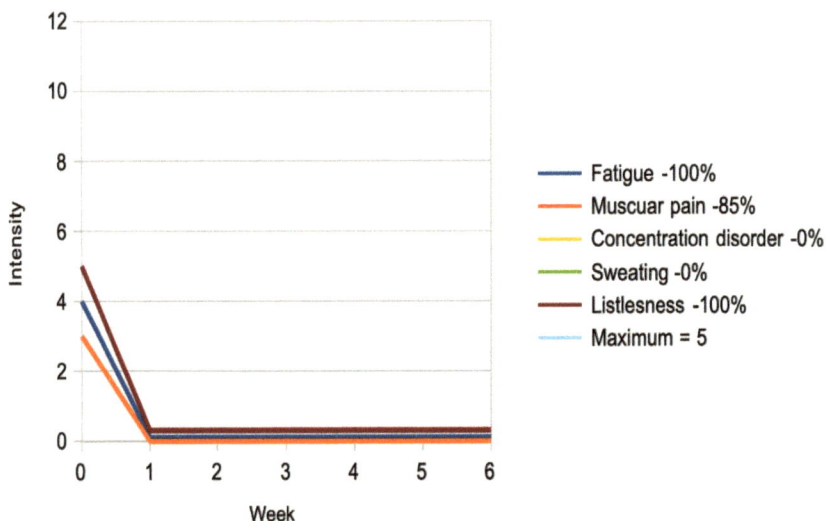

Time of the interviews: 6 weeks after the end of the first combination therapy, at the beginning of relapse therapy, and after 3 weeks of combination therapy

Comment: about 3-4 weeks after several flu-like infections, the symptoms of an active toxoplasmosis appeared, which increased over some months. The time of the toxoplasmosis infection remains unclear, but the toxoplasmosis IgG was above the test's measuring range after a disease duration of 7 months.   Despite the typical toxoplasmosis symptoms, the IgM value was not positive. The therapy worked quickly and effectively. At the end of January 2017, Ms S. was free from symptoms and she still was in December, 2018.

Addition in 10/2019:

In 6/2019 Ms S. suffered from another relapse, which did not come as a sur-prise, given that her Toxoplasma IgG had been elevated beyond measurement (above 400 IU/ml) before the first treatment in 8/2016, while the IgM was only slightly, not significantly elevated at 4,75 AU/ml.   In 6/2019, the LTT had already been established in my daily work, and so we estimated it along with the Toxoplasma antibodies. The Toxoplasma LTT was 89,3 SI (positive: above 3), while the IgG was elevated at 106 IU/ml, the IgM was below the measure range of 3 AU/ml.

Case 1 (pp 84-87) corresponds to this observation. In 7/2019 Ms M. suffered from a relapse, the Toxoplasma IgG was rated 12,4 IU/ml (17,5 IU/ml before the first treatment), the IgM was negative (as before the first treatment), the Toxoplasma LTT showed, at 16,2 SI, a significant positive result.

Another   corresponding result of the Toxoplasma LTT could be verified in case 7 of the original case compilation. Before the first treatment in 1/2016 the IgG rated at 37,9 AU/ml, the IgM at 3,99 AU/ml. When a relapse occurred in 7/2019 Toxoplasma IgG was 18,9 IU/ml, the IgM below measurable. The Toxoplasma checklist indicated at a high risk for an chronic active toxoplasmosis, the LTT was rated 8,5 SI. The treatment showed again a very positive result.

Considered, that in all three cases the tachyzoite-specific IgG has decreased in comparison to the previous treatment, while the IgM had been negative or turned to negative, there has obviously been no renewed activity of tachyzoites. It can be assumed, that the the symptoms in all three cases - as well as the elevated Toxoplasma LTT's - are a result of renewed bradyzoite activity, because as   has been stated before: Bradyzoite activity cannot be revealed by tachyzoite-specific IgG and IgM assays. During a toxoplasmosis treatment of 4 weeks the symptoms of all three patients vanished completely.

10.1. Cases without antibody detection

After the case of Ms S, with the highest Toxoplasma antibody value, 5 cases will be presented which were completely negative on Toxoplasma IgG and IgM tests. These patients nevertheless suffered from the same symptoms as the ones presented in the previous cases, and the toxoplasmosis therapy proved to be even more effective. This still evokes my colleagues´ incomprehension, but these cases are *not in contradiction to basic research* (see pages 36, 37). I know that I am repeating myself, but in short:

If an infection with Toxoplasma gondii has occurred a longer time ago, the detectable antibodies, which can exclusively record the fast form of Toxoplasma, the *tachyzoites*, slowly decrease. After some years, they cannot be detected anymore.   Please take note, that it never has been investigated, how long antibodies last after a primary infection. If the immune system becomes exhausted by the Toxoplasma or weakened by a different disease, a *reactivation* of the Toxoplasma can take place and the activity slowly increases. This initially happens mainly inside their cysts in the form of *bradyzoites*, the activity of which we cannot detect with currently used antibody assays, as these have been designed to detect tachyzoite – specific antibodies.

> *Toxoplasma doesn't lose the ability to multiply after having changed to bradyzoites (84), and it has been proven that bradyzoite - activity can cause significant symptoms (42). We cannot assume that such activity would leave our health unaffected, but we do know, that Toxoplasma activity can result in elevation of cytokine – levels (27), and these are known to mediate inflammation.*

An increased tachyzoite activity would only be detectable if a massive conversion of bradyzoites to tachyzoites took place, and if these would then erupt from their host cells and induce a renewed antibody production. The patients listed here showed the same symptoms of an active toxoplasmosis as the patients with a positive toxoplasmosis IgG in the first group, and the treatment was even more effective. Even a complete lack of antibody detection as in group B is no contradiction to recent research. To my knowledge the reliability of antibody assays has never been proven for Toxoplasma reactivation, which can take place years after the initial infection and then cause a chronic disease.

In my talks with professors at two universities, as well as in discussions with colleagues it is pointed out that placebo effects might be the reason for improvement. Please read the case studies and judge for yourself if a patient who is so seriously ill can be treated effectively by a placebo effect. After having acquired 25 years of professional experience, I would rule that out. Recent personal experience concerning the toxoplasma LTT is encouraging (see pp. 212 - 220), but it is not perfect, and it will only be widely accepted after it has been evaluated in a clinical study.

The new methods which at the time are being developed (see p. 209 - 211) might also play an important part in future Toxoplasma diagnostics, but these have to undergo an evaluation as well. The mills of medicine research grind slowly, but extremely carefully and there is no doubt that we want it that way. The disadvantage is that this takes a lot of time, and some patients are far too ill to wait until a test which can detect bradyzoite activity in *every* case might be accessible in some years. *We might have to re-think and act earlier.*

Case 19, Ms Julia S., age 25

Since approximately one and a half years, Ms S. had been suffering from unclear, slowly increasing bouts of sweating, which brought her to my practice in January, 2015. All laboratory values and ultrasound examinations remained inconspicuous and no further examinations were carried out on the otherwise fit and resilient student. One year later Ms S. came to my practice again. She felt considerably worse and complained about severe bouts of sweating, unclear tachycardia and swelling of the cervical lymph nodes. Erythrocyte sedimentation was increased at 46/66 mm, the CRP (an inflammation value) was increased to 2.7 mg/dl (normal is 0.5 mg/dl).

Furthermore, several liver values were increased significantly and the ultrasound revealed an enlarged spleen. Antibodies against the Epstein-Barr virus (EBV, see page 63) were significantly increased, indicating clearly that glandular fever, synonymous with an acute mononucleosis was persisting at that time. EBV is a viral infection which usually heals on its own within a few weeks.

Under care her physical condition and the laboratory values returned back to normal by March of 2016 and Ms S. was able to engage in physical exertion again. But then, in September, 2016, she suffered from 3 successive severe infections within a few weeks accompanied by an unclear weakening, resulting in her coming to my practice again in November, 2016. Further inquiries revealed that she had not only been suffering from increased sweating for about 2 years, but also from other symptoms. These were muscular pain, fatigue, concentration disorders, joint pains, a generalized physical weakness and morning stiffness.

She had also noticed dyspnoea and tachycardia at even light exertion, as well as a frequent, severe dizziness and a frequent swelling of the cervical lymph nodes prior to her EBV infection.

The December 2016 blood count, blood sedimentation, all liver values, vitamin D and iron storage were normal. The EBV IgG was significantly increased at 433 U/ml (positive is above 20) and the IgM was negative. This is typical for an elapsed EBV infection.

The Toxoplasma IgG was negative, IgM 3.7 AU/l. At that time the symptoms had been increasingly persistent for about 2 years, and two months before, a considerable worsening had started. As mentioned several times previously, an active toxoplasmosis cannot be safely ruled out by antibody values, especially if numerous toxoplasmosis symptoms are combined, as was the case here.

Therapy: Clindamycine 300 3x1 was prescribed. This led to a considerable improvement of many symptoms in the course of 11 days, however the bouts of sweating, morning stiffness, listlessness and irritability initially remained unaffected. Daraprim, calcium folinate and sulfadiazine were prescribed, which initially led to an improvement. After 20 days, sulfadiazine was stopped due to a decreasing effectiveness and clindamycin 300 3x1, Daraprim and calcium folinate were combined instead. As a consequence, the remaining symptoms were also reduced to 0, so that the therapy could be stopped after 30 days altogether.

Ms S.: results and improvement of symptoms in %

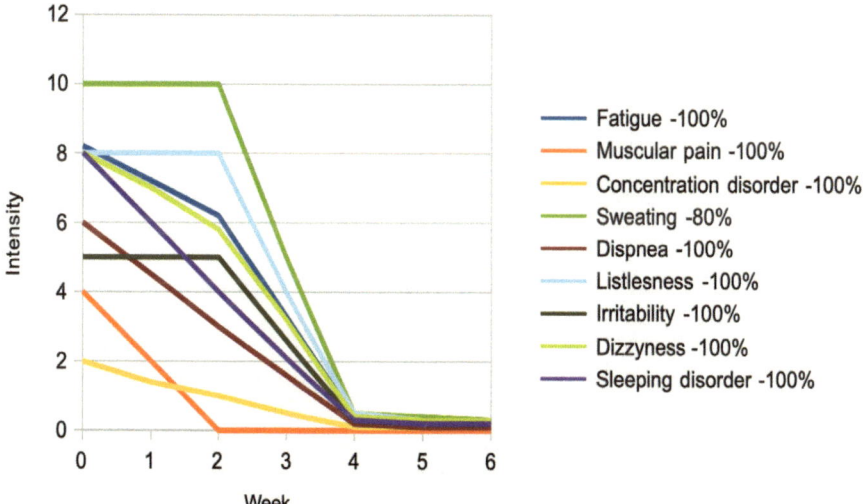

Time of the interviews: prior to therapy, after 11 days of Clindamycine 300 3x1, and after 4 weeks of combination therapy

Comment: The mononucleosis lasted from January to March 2016 and weakened the patient. From September, 2016 frequent infections and increasing symptoms of an active toxoplasmosis, which had probably been persisting before, appeared. There are many patients who suffer from a chronic fatigue syndrome (CFS) following mononucleosis.

This case shows that a mononucleosis can weaken the immune system in a way, that a hitherto pre-existing toxoplasmosis might enter into a more active stage. Since in some CFS patients, the disease is started by a mononucleosis, this could be an explanation for their CFS. This corresponds with basic research, such cases have been describe earlier (45). In October 2019 Ms S. is still free from symptoms.

Case 21, Ms Iris H., age 35

Ms H. gave birth to a healthy son in 2009 and to a healthy daughter in 2012. After the second birth, she recovered only very slowly. She was frequently tired and worn out, had nocturnal bouts of sweating and became very nervous and irritable. A postnatal depression was diagnosed.

A slowly increasing dyspnoea and increased tachycardia developed at the same time and even regular stair climbing caused problems for Ms H. Considerable water retention in the lower legs, as well as morning stiffness and muscular pains also occurred and she sometimes felt very weak. Every now and then a blurred vision occurred, without an apparent cause. These symptoms showed a slow, but continuously increasing tendency over about 3 ½ years.

In December, 2016 tests for Toxoplasma IgG and IgM were negative. The patient had been ill for approximately 5 years. As seen in the previous case, a chronic active toxoplasmosis could not be ruled out based on laboratory values without considering observed symptoms.

Therapy: With typical clinical symptoms for an active toxoplasmosis a therapeutic trial with clindamycin 2 x 600 mg was carried out. This led to a slight improvement of the tiredness in particular, as well as muscular pains, so that from the beginning of 2017 a combination therapy with clindamycin, Daraprim and sulfadiazine was prescribed. Now all symptoms improved continuously and the treatment could be stopped after one month.

Ms I.H.: results and improvement of symptoms in %

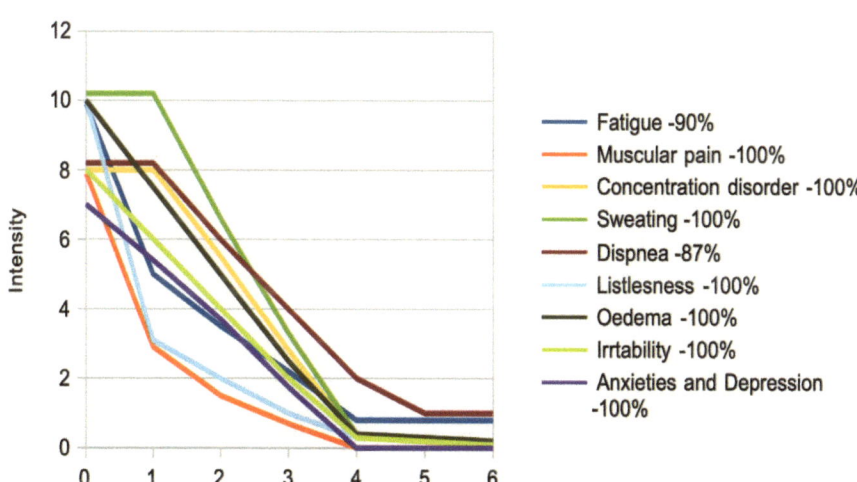

Time of the interviews: prior to therapy, after one week clindamycine 600 2x1, after 4 weeks of combination therapy

In addition to the changes shown in the graphic, visual disturbances were reduced from 3 to 0, and sleeping disorder, upper abdominal symptoms and the diffuse feeling of pressure in the abdomen were reduced from 10 to 0.

Comment: a depressive progression at the end of pregnancy seamlessly transitioned to an active toxoplasmosis, the symptoms of which slowly but continuously increased over a period of 8 years. A similar development had taken place in case 23 also. **These cases show, that it is advisable to consider an active toxoplasmosis as cause of the disease in case of a lengthy postnatal depression, and to specifically ask about these symptoms.**

141

Case 24, Ms Regina H., age 45

In September, 2012, Ms H. fell ill from pneumonia, from which she did not recover well. A dyspnoea at even the slightest exertion remained for months and therefore Ms H. was transferred for a cardiological examination. That discovered a reduced pumping function of the left heart chamber, which is doing the main work. A heart catheter examination was carried out which showed that the coronary vessels were not constricted; no cause for the dyspnoea was found.

A follow-up cardiological examination was carried out in July, 2013, which yielded no changes to the preliminary findings. A pulmonary medical examination in December found nothing.

In October of the next year, another cardiological examination was carried out because of a dyspnoea with sweating, which showed unchanged normal results. A full two years after the pneumonia, a severe limitation of heart-circulation resilience was still persisting, without a detectable reason.

Ms H. now reported that she had been suffering from increasing concentration disorders since mid-2015, and since the beginning of 2016 she experienced a profound depression. Her husband explained that his wife had been nervous and lacked concentration, and she sometimes cried without any obvious reason. According to her own judgement, Ms H. was lacking all vitality and interest in life. From about March of 2016, generalized muscular pains and sweating, which also continuously increased, had also occurred. **In September of 2016 the Toxoplasma IgG and IgM were negative. At that time the symptoms had been persisting for about 4 years.**

Therapy: after receiving suitable information, I prescribed clindamycin 2 x 600 mg. Within one week muscular pains and tiredness improved considerably, and concentration disorders and sweating decreased slightly. A combination therapy with Daraprim, calcium folinate and sulfadiazine was prescribed, under which all symptoms improved considerably, so that the therapy could be stopped after 4 weeks. By January, 2017 the symptoms had been in remission for about 3 months.

Ms R.H.: results and improvement of symptoms in %

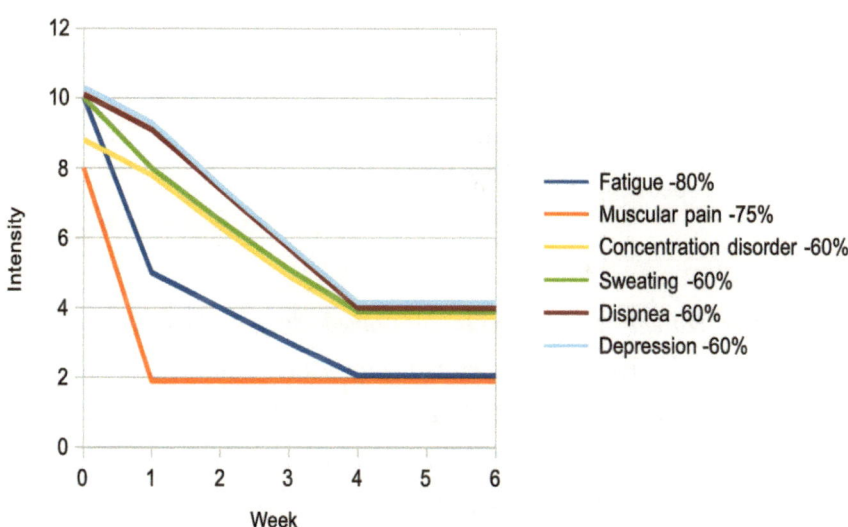

Time of the interviews: prior to therapy, after one week clindamycine 600 2x1, and after 4 weeks combination therapy

Comment: a pneumonia in September of 2012 probably led to an increase in activity of a pre-existing toxoplasmosis, however the initial infection had taken place such a long time ago that antibodies could not be detected any more.

The dyspnoea that started in October 2012 was a first symptom for toxoplasmosis and repeated cardiologic and pulmonary examinations showed a reduced ejection fraction (EF) of the heart of 45%, without a discernible reason found.

This is the only case, in which dyspnoea and later concentration disorder in combination with depressive moods preceded muscular pains. *After the toxoplasmosis treatment the EF increased to a normal value of 55%,* and the exertinonal dyspnoea was improved considerably. Possibly, a prolonged therapy could have yielded an even better result, although the patient was very content with the result of the therapy, and thus it was stopped. Ms H. experienced only very few side-effects and would repeat the therapy if necessary.

The patient quite literally blossomed during therapy, showed a renewed vitality, recuperated physically and could leave her depressive moods behind. That is a wonderful sight and as a doctor, one is simply very happy and thankful for a positive development like that. That just has to be said here.

Case 25, Mr Paul T., age 57

Mr T. is a younger looking, athletic patient, who has been exclusively eating vegan food for about three years. Since about 1990 he has nursed diseased cats for several years, and since 1992, an unclear rapid fatigue as well as unclear sweating, joint pains and an unusual sensitivity to cold had been persisting.

All laboratory values, antibodies against anaplasma (a bacterium from tick bites), borreliosis, specialized rheumatism values (CCP, ANA, AMA, Waaler-Rose test) and a blood protein test (electrophoresis) were negative, as were several tumour markers (CEA, Ca19-9 and PSA). The values for an inflammation of the liver (hepatitis B and C) as well as a HIV-test were negative. Only the hepatitis A IgG was slightly increased, which showed that Mr T. had gone through a light liver inflammation in the past. In January, 2007 a gallbladder removal was performed, however, this improved the physical condition slightly.

A catheter examination of the bile duct and the pancreas (ERCP) was done three years later. In March, 2011 a bilateral thyroid removal was performed due to nodes.

During a brief interview in my practice in November, 2016, Mr T.´s overall physical condition was mentioned. He had been feeling very exhausted for years, "like a candle that was burning on both ends", was unbalanced, had severe bouts of sweating, suffered from morning stiffness, but had not talked about it for a long time, since he had attributed that condition primarily to his heavy occupational burden and had become accustomed to it.

We went through the Toxoplasma-checklist and a high risk for an active toxoplasmosis was indicated. Already several extensive examinations had been carried out in the past and thus any another disease could be virtually ruled out. **The November, 2016 Toxoplasma check showed high probability for toxoplasmosis with negative laboratory findings for Toxoplasma, borreliosis, CCP; inconspicuous blood values and normal blood sedimentation. Symptoms had persisted for about 24 years.**

Therapy: A therapy with Daraprim, calcium folinate and sulfadiazine was prescribed, which led to a very significant improvement of *all* symptoms within 10 days.

On January 3rd, 2017 medication was stopped due to suspected side-effects and laboratory values were checked. Apart from a moderate increase in liver value (GGT) and a slight decrease of white blood cells to 3400/ul (normal from 4200/ul), normal values were found.

Since the result of the therapy had been very good to then, a cessation of therapy was agreed to, and from January 4th, the side effects ceased and about 3-4 days later he was almost free from symptoms.

Unfortunately, all previous symptoms slowly reappeared within two weeks. A combination therapy with clindamycin 600 2x1 instead of sulfadiazine was prescribed and this led to an alleviation of all symptoms within 3 days. The therapy was carried out for one month and could be successfully stopped then.

Mr T.: results and improvement of symptoms in %

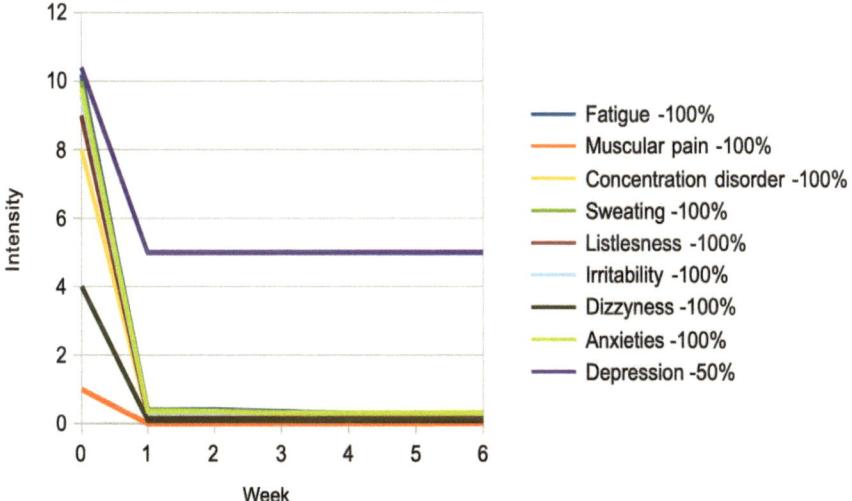

Comment: the therapy had to be stopped with a very good treatment success after 12 days due to side effects. The symptoms intensified again quickly. Due to the Christmas holidays, when that phase took place, there is sadly no documentation of the therapy setback, and the healing process was less streamline than the graphic suggests. After 2 weeks, a continuation of the therapy with a changed combination was necessary, which again was very effective. Therefore, we can conclude that in clinical pictures with long disease durations it is necessary to carry out a therapy for at least one months, regardless of a rapid efficacy.

By the end of January of 2017, Mr T. had been free from symptoms for about three weeks. The result of the first week of treatment was unusually positive. In this case the patient had been prescribed a combination therapy right from the start upon his own express request.

The graphic representation reaches its limit here. The symptom intensity of 10 had been noted for fatigue, sweating, irritability, anxiety and depression, and since all these symptom intensities have been reduced to 0 quickly, the according graphs overlap completely. I had to separate the graphs to make each of them visible.

Mr T. has written a protocol about his illness and the therapy, and they are quite informative.

Toxoplasmosis-diary of Mr T. 12/2016:

"For over 20 years, stiffness of gait, constant fatigue with very little recreative sleep, frightening nightmares, morning anxiety, depressive moods, aggression and overreactions, at times provocative risk-taking have been persisting. The sense of smell is impaired, weak scents cannot be perceived. Due to an extreme daytime fatigue a strong need to sleep is felt. Quick gripping and coordinative motions are sloppy, the hand-eye coordination has decreased considerably. This is especially noticeable while playing darts, at tennis or playing the guitar.

A severe nocturnal sweating persists, up to 6 times nocturnal urination with dripping of urine, dry mouth in the morning. The short-term memory is impaired and word-finding disturbances occur, names cannot be remembered, appointments are often "forgotten" and much more.

An agonizing listlessness and joint pains persist, (and) for safety reasons because of a muscular weakness, stairs are descended while being turned backwards. Despite being able to carry out physically demanding chores a feeling of decreasing physical capacity exists, but rarely muscular pains. Significantly longer regeneration times are needed. In irregular intervals a light, pulling – unpleasant feeling located near the liver is felt, simultaneously to a pulling pain in the area of the heart left (independent from strain, consumption of alcohol...) in some situation the feeling of cold triggers an almost uncontrollable, chill-like symptoms, which disappears after about 5 minutes without any consequences.

Start of therapy with Daraprim 2x1, calcium folinate 1x1, sulfadiazine 4x1

Monday, 19/12/2016: in the evening 7 p.m. initial dose; at 10 p.m. slight change in visual acuity (peripheral vision sharper), nocturnal sleep slightly deeper than usual

20/12/2016: after getting up, the usual morning stiffness of gait was almost gone completely, a normal level of activity can be achieved faster, no more low point in the course of the day.

21/12/2016: at work almost suddenly knowledge of all names of colleagues. Nocturnal sleep deep and free from dreams, lesser nocturnal waking phases and visits to the toilet.

22/12/2016: Night spent more quietly, getting up is almost free from problems, no low point during daytime, the improvement of the memory for names continues. The flickering eyesight with longer reading decreases. Hearing is more precise and more selective. The frequent urge to pass urine and the dripping have decreased significantly.

Note: In 2017 it was shown that Toxoplasma can also cause an inflammation of the prostate (13); this would explain the frequent urge to pass urine and the dripping prior to therapy and the vanishing of these symptoms after the toxoplasmosis therapy.

23/12/2016: This has been the first complete night of undisturbed sleep for years!!! Deep and without nightmares, no visit to the toilet. I have the impression of being faster, the gripping security has increased significantly. I am much calmer at work.

24/12/2016: The night's sleep has been very good again, there were no more nightmares, morning anxiety is only minimal and decreasing. The forefoot-strike is almost back to normal, the numbness in the toes decreasing to vanishing. The work efficiency is significantly higher, more precise work with smaller tools is possible without problems.

25/12/2016: I wanted to lie down during daytime and tried to sleep for half an hour, but that was not possible, since I am not tired anymore. Playing the guitar and darts have become much easier.

26/12/2016: A strange day. All past symptoms appear again in reverse order – deep sleep at noon, I feel restless. The elbows and sometimes the knees hurt. It seems as if my body would run through all the stages in fast-forward mode.

27/12/2016: Slept well. No more urological problems for days, the scent of the urine is now normal. Stools are normal as well. The body now expresses an enormous pent-up demand for recreation and sleep. The feeling of hunger has changed, I don't feel like eating so much anymore, and my craving for sweets has decreased significantly.

28/12/2016: Slept deep and without dreams or significant interruptions. The manual skills have improved, planning ability is better, work is approached in a more consequent way and finished. Forgetfulness has been reduced considerably, very little irritability or open anger.

29/12/2016: A very successful day (technically), but I am also very tired. Yet the tiredness is not unpleasant. The days also feel longer, there is "more time".

From the 30/12/2016 side-effects can be increasingly felt: joint pains, severe nocturnal sweating, nausea, light headaches, occasional dizziness, pulling pains round the kidneys, weakness, chills, fainting.

03/01/2017: In the doctor's practice the medication was stopped at once and blood samples were taken.

04/01/2017: The side-effects start to decrease.

18/01/2017: Restart of therapy with changed combination, now good tolerance of medication. Significant reduction of all symptoms after about three days; this time the treatment is carried out for 4 weeks.

What remained positive:

Without the nocturnal visits to the toilet, I can sleep well and restful through the night, there are no more morning stiffness or joint pains, no morning anxieties and the depressive moods are decreasing considerably. I can laugh again! There is still some daytime tiredness, but the sleep is more recreative now.   I have a huge pent-up demand for sleep and I can sleep undisturbed for 10-12 hours at the moment. The motor skills are increasing visibly, the muscles are generally stronger, there are no more muscular pains. The pains around the liver and the heart do not occur anymore. I don't have cravings anymore, the appetite for a combination of sweets and alcohol is gone. I have a significantly better feeling in the balls of the feet and in the toes."

Case 26, Ms. Yasemin U., age 42

Ms U. reported that she had been feeling weak and with very little resiliency for years and she often felt dizzy. An examination of the equilibrium organ yielded a normal result. A neurological examination and a nuclear spin examination of the head were inconspicuous.

In November, 2011 a severe vitamin D deficiency was detected. After high-dosage administration of 20.000 units daily for 50 days, the symptom improved slightly.

In mid-2015 the dizziness increased, and headaches in the back of the head, a pronounced light-sensitivity of the eyes and visual disorders occurred, lasting for days. Since autumn 2015, increased sweating occurred and after New Year's, 2016 Ms U. had been increasingly tired and listless and she was constantly experiencing a severe urge to sleep.

In March, 2016, a significant, unclear increase in weight took place, accompanied by increased loss of hair, shivering, increase of dizziness (rated 9) and sleep disorders (8). A thyroid disorder and a thyroid insufficiency were excluded, and the inflammation value, blood count and examination of the blood proteins were inconspicuous.

A month later an increased dyspnoea and tachycardia at even light physical exertion developed and noticeable water retention in the lower legs appeared. In combination these symptoms are alarming with regards to a possible heart insufficiency. A diuretic (Torasemid 10mg 1x daily) slightly improved the symptoms, but I transferred the patient to a cardiological unit as soon as possible to clarify the causes. Only a slight thickening of the heart muscle with normal pumping capacity, as well as a minor pericardial effusion were diagnosed.

During stress ECG the patient was resilient up to 75 W, yet she experienced a beginning dyspnoea at even this comparatively low strain and her heart frequency at 160 beats per minute was clearly increased too much compared to the strain. This is similar to the cases 1, 5, 6 and 16. A heart insufficiency II°-III° and a chronic pericarditis (water retention in the pericardium) were diagnosed, but without a reason being found. The ECG showed changes in the sense of a possible circulatory disorder of the coronary vessels, but a coronary angiography (heart catheter examination) and the laboratory values yielded normal results.

In September, 2016 the Toxoplasma checklist showed a high risk for an active toxoplasmosis with a negative IgG and IgM. The symptoms had been persisting for about 20 years altogether, and they had considerably worsened within the last 5 years.

Therapy: clindamycin 600mg 2x1 was prescribed. Within one week some symptoms improved considerably, but the therapy was not continued by the patient due to family problems. Within 3 days the symptoms returned to full intensity.

In October, 2016 clindamycin 2 x 600mg was prescribed again. After 3 weeks of clindamycin administration the symptoms had improved very well. Ms U. nevertheless felt a slight increase in muscular pains and sweating again. Now the treatment was continued with a combination therapy of Daraprim, calcium folinate and sulfadiazine for 4 weeks, which was completed successfully.

Ms U.: results and improvement of symptoms in %

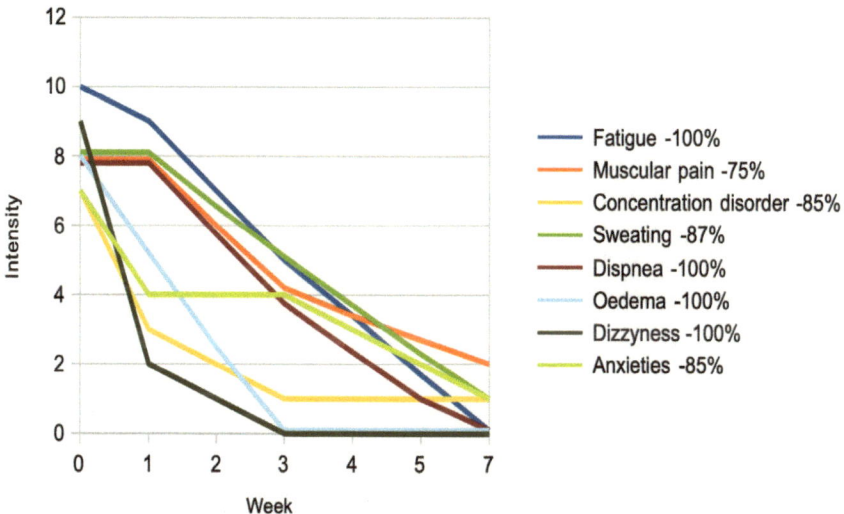

Time of the interviews: prior to therapy, after 1 and 3 weeks of clindamycine 600 2x1 and after 4 weeks combination therapy

Comment: symptoms, which could later be attributed to an active toxoplasmosis, had been persisting for about 20 years, but had increased within the last 5 years. In April, 2016 a further significant worsening with an increase in dyspnoea, water retention and weight gain occurred. This was diagnosed as a medium-grade heart insufficiency NYHA II°-III°, without a discernible reason found. This problem was eliminated completely by the toxoplasmosis therapy and the diuretic could be stopped. This was the patient with the most severe cardio-vascular/lung-impairment because of an active toxoplasmosis.

The patient is still free from symptoms and resilient again.

11. Results

A scientific work generally presents the results in a separate chapter and conclusions are then drawn in a different chapter for "discussion". This practice mostly constitutes a very "dry" result section, which is not very appealing to the reader. I have compiled a summarized version of both sections. Those who are looking for more scientific details and who are missing the "dry stuff" may review my original work on pages 83 to 90 and the discussion on pages 93 to 112. That will surely be reasonably "dry".

First of all, and far from self-evident so far, my findings indicate that the "Toxoplasma-load" of an immunocompetent person, that is somebody with an intact immune system, can be active and can trigger severe chronic symptoms in the sense of a chronic active toxoplasmosis (see references 22, 28, 29, 30, 31, 42, 83).

The clinical picture is presented in detail on pages 56 to 60 as well as in the case studies. The severe symptoms, which mostly increased in the course of years, impaired the affected patients seriously, but were often categorized as "sore muscles", "stress", "afflictions of age", "poor physical condition", "wear and tear" or "unclear depressions". There is also progression in intervals, that is, phases with few symptoms alternating with acute episodes (cases 8, 11, 13, 16, 23).

This impedes a speedy diagnose and has to be questioned in greater detail during anamnesis (anamnesis is Doctor-speak for "gathering the patient's history"). I always ask my patients to specify their symptoms according to their "bad days" when working with the checklist.

I assume that the immune system of these patients gains the upper hand in the phases when they have few symptoms, which can extend from days to sometimes 2-3 weeks.

Unfortunately, that success is not lasting, and in the end the disease is sadly just "almost" under control, and the person is chronically ill. According to my experience, the diagnose of an active toxoplasmosis with progression in intervals is more difficult to work out, but in exchange this form can generally be treated very well (cases 8, 11, 13, 16 and 23). It seems to be easier in these cases to move the jittery balance between our immune system and the parasite in our favour.

The disease durations observed in the case studies vary from 7 months up to 50 years, which is a huge span. This can completely scatter entire life-plans of the affected. On average, the disease durations of group A with a positive IgG antibody detection was 10 years and that of group B without antibody detection 5.8 years.

A constant problem in the anamneses is that the onset of the disease is slow and insidious in most cases, so that a clear beginning of the illness and clear symptoms can be defined only with difficulty at the beginning, and that these indications to an active toxoplasmosis can be misinterpreted by the patient as well as the doctor as an age - related, though strongly increasing health complaint. Therefore, the disease might not be noticed as such at the beginning, and a time period for the illness is hard to determine.

It is conceivable that in very long disease durations also patients of the second group might develop antibodies again. That would be the time from which the immune system has become so weakened that Toxoplasma can again increasingly flood the organism in the form of tachyzoites. Not a desirable development! It is also remarkable that in both groups the effectiveness of the immune system is impaired by an active toxoplasmosis. Several patients reported strikingly frequent infections (viral infections as well as infections of the skin) and these occurred considerably less often or not at all after a toxoplasmosis therapy.

11.1. Women are affected frequently

Astoundingly, there are only 6 male patients among the 27 patients of the case studies, even though it was proven in 2016 that in Germany Toxoplasma antibodies are 1.76 times more frequently found in men than in women (88). This is an ongoing trend in my daily practice, and I continue to identify more women than men with this clinical picture. Possible explanations would be that health-related problems are on average less-frequently addressed by men and/or are considered to be signs of age-related ailments or symptoms of wear and tear, and are thus not talked about.

> *This reinforces the need for a structured interview, for example by using a checklist. Patients usually give their physician detailed information about their complaints, but sometimes crucial information is left out. We need to ask them the right questions.*

11.2. Antibody detection in younger patients is less frequent

The median age of 59 years (range 35 - 82) of the 17 patients of group A with antibody detection is 16 years higher than that of the 10 patients of group B without antibody detection, where the median age is 43 years (range 25 - 57). It is known that the frequency of positive Toxoplasma antibody detection in the overall population increases with age (49, 88). This has been discussed in detail under 6.3., pp. 47 / 48. Therefore, it doesn't come as a surprise that the IgG antibody detection of the patients of group A, who are on average older, is positive, but why is that so?

The first logical explanation at hand might be that in a longer span of life the Toxoplasma simply have more time to cause an infection. It can also be argued that after a primary infection, it might be only a matter of time or an eventual weakening of the immune system that toxoplasma get the chance to crank up their metabolism, transform to tachyzoits, blast their host cells and then appear again, after many years, in the bloodstream. Such a spreading of parasites can possibly take place at a older age in correlation with a longer disease duration and an exhaustion of the immune system a long time after the initial infection, and can then lead to a measurable increase in tachyzoite antibodies.

With regards to the completely "antibody negative" patients of group B, who on average are younger, it has been shown in several studies that Toxoplasma can be present in an organism despite negative antibody detection (24, 53, 94). This suggests that some humans carry Toxoplasma without it being detectable at the moment. Thankfully, this only results in an illness in some of these carriers.

If an increase of Toxoplasma activity takes place without tachyzoites breaking free from cysts, the antibody assays will still render negative results. The disease is then caused predominantly by bradyzoite activity, and basic research shows this is absolutely possible (42). Bradyzoites don't rest peacefully.

The sensitivity of Toxoplasma IgM and IgG assays in case of a reactivation of Toxoplasma activity in humans with normal immune system has never been investigated or proven. In my experience I have come to the conclusion, that antibody assays are very unreliable when the disease is caused predominantly by a slowly increasing Toxoplasma activity within the cysts in the course of a chronic active toxoplasmosis.

The number of Toxoplasma carriers without detectable tachyzoites antibodies, who can potentially become ill from a chronic active toxoplasmosis based on an increased activity within the cysts is unclear. From my observations it can be assumed that the number is significant, otherwise there would not appear so many younger patients in my case collection (about 40%), who suffer from a chronic active toxoplasmosis without any detectable tachyzoite antibodies.

11.3. Significance of antibody detection

For a better understanding of the following explanations it is important to initially clarify the limits of our current laboratory medicine again:

> *Tests only react to tachyzoite-specific antibodies and the sensitivity of a standard test system in case of an initial infection is only 81.8% (65). Basic research has done further substantial work which questions the accuracy of Toxoplasma antibody assays. "The currently available solid phase immunoassays were developed in the 1970's to detect strains which were circulating at that time" and there are strong indications, that.. (..) ..standard assays may substantially underestimate the prevalence of Toxoplasma infection in a population and its effect on health and disease" (93).*

> *Further it has been proven that, in cases of a Toxoplasma infection, tachyzoite-specific IgG, IgM and even PCR can render negative results (24, 46, 53). In a chronic active course of the disease, reliability of our currently used lab methods has not been proven and these are most likely not suitable to detect Bradyzoites or their activity, let alone the cyst burden.*

Only the 17 patients in Group A had detectable Toxoplasma IgG values, and these ranged from a low of 20 to a high of 400+ (above the ability of the test to measure), a huge range. If tachyzoit activity were relevant in the presented cases, there should be a correlation between symptom ratings and IgG values (or IgM, if they were present), with lower values associated with less severe symptoms and higher values with more severe symptoms. *That correlation is not apparent.*

For example the symptoms in case 5 with a disease duration of 50 years are very pronounced; nevertheless Toxoplasma IgG antibodies were increased only moderate at 32,5 IU/ml, the IgM was negative. This case can most likely be compared with cases 14 and 16, still the IgG values (with similar negative IgM) for these patients had been more than thrice increased. The equally severe cases 21 and 26 of group B could be consulted as comparison as well, the antibody detections of which were completely negative.

> *These observations show that the level of tachyzoite-specific IgG doesn't allow any conclusions with regards to the intensity of chronic active toxoplasmosis, if they can be determined at all. Since I assume that the reason for my patients' illness can be found in the intensive activity inside the bradyzoite cysts, it is explainable that a correlation between the intensity of the disease and the available laboratory values cannot be seen here.*

The detection of IgG values indicating the presence of antibodies occurs with symptoms, but the reverse is not necessarily true. The presence of symptoms does not indicate the presence of antibodies. *Since a significant IgM increase could not be found in any case in either Group A or B, a secure exclusion of a chronic active toxoplasmosis is clearly not possible by determination of the tachyzoite-specific IgM.*

The current medical opinion is still that a negative IgM excludes an active toxoplasmosis and thus the need of a therapy. Due to research having hinted repeatedly of a significant effect of bradyzoite activity, and due to my own observations, I definitely cannot agree with that.

Research still focuses predominantely on acute rather than chronic toxoplasmosis and it is only a general assumption, that cases with chronically active courses of the disease as presented here could be diagnosed by using the usual antibody assays - to my knowledge this has never been proven.

Just to clarify it unmistakably: From my point of view, the unwavering belief in the significance of tachyzoite-specific antibody values is, at least with regards to chronic active toxoplasmosis, a fatal error of medicine.

The 10 patients of group B are on average 16 years younger than Group A patients and their disease duration is about 4 years shorter at 5.8 years compared to patients of group A. In group B, neither Toxoplasma IgM nor Toxoplasma IgG were detectable. I see the reason for that in the more active immune system of the younger patients, which severely attacks Toxoplasma at an early stage, so that the parasites have to retreat into cysts as bradyzoites to survive. This probably reduces the trigger for antibody production at an early stage, since Toxoplasma in the form of tachyzoites are then not "visible" to the immune system anymore.

It can be furthermore assumed, that Toxoplasma did not exhaust the immune system of these patients so much since they were on average younger, fitter and the disease duration was somewhat shorter. As long as the immune system is adequately active, Toxoplasma have to remain in their cysts to survive and cannot be present in the blood. In that form they do not cause a renewed formation of tachyzoite antibodies, which could then be detected with our tests.

If the immune system ceases to produce Tachyzoite antibodies after some years, the disease will no longer be detectable in the blood. This does not mean that the Toxoplasma in the cysts are inactive. There are numerous indications that an increased activity in the cysts can trigger a symptomatic illness, since, contrary to older assumptions, *bradyzoites do not rest*, but can be active and can reproduce and cause illness. This refers to the findings of Fergusson et al. (1989), McLeod et al. (2008) and Watts et al. (2015) (26, 42, 84).

I am convinced that a significant activity within the cysts, predominantly of the bradyzoites, is the decisive reason for the illness in both groups of patients who all have inconspicuous IgM values with regards to tachyzoites, and whose IgG values, if indeed there are any, don't show any direct correlation to the severity of the illness. The clinical pictures in both groups are identical, and the toxoplasmosis therapy is even more effective in group B.

The bradyzoites, the activity of which we cannot measure, are currently underrated strongly, and our established laboratory values produce only a pretended security. It is difficult to develop reliable bradyzoite-specific tests, since bradyzoites reveal themselves only rarely to the immune system and only lead to a limited antibody production (76).

Thankfully, basic research has begun to address this problem, and there are new and promising methods being developed, with the aim of getting a grip on this problem and reveal hitherto not detectable toxoplasma presence and even to determine the cyst burden (93). See also chapter 14 beginning on page 209.

11.4. The frequency of a chronic active toxoplasmosis

If one relates the 27 presented cases to my average of 1250 patients per quarter, a frequency of 2.1% can be assumed. Yet, during the documentation of my observations during the last three years while I was writing this book and working on the the translation, a lot of cases of an active toxoplasmosis came to light, and the real frequency in my practice will therefore be significantly higher.

Possibly, there are also more male patients with an active toxoplasmosis in my practice, who simply have not been "caught" due to the reasons mentioned on page 145. It also needs to be considered that the rate of infestation in the east of Germany is on average 20% higher than in the west of Germany. It also follows that more patients are suffering from an active toxoplasmosis there. Our practice is located in North Rhine-Westphalia, i.e. in the west of Germany.

Addition in 10/2019: Until now I have treated well over 150 patients who suffered from chronic active toxoplasmosis (including some patients who have been referred from colleagues), and since February 2019 there are many among them, in which a chronic active toxoplasmosis was confirmed not only by a successful treatment, but by a positive Toxoplasma LTT as well. (see pages 211 - 220)

> *If one calculates very conservatively with only about 25 cases of active toxoplasmosis per general practitioner in Germany (recently about 83,000,000 inhabitants and 32,600 licensed general practitioners) this results in about 81,000 persons or about 1% of the overall population who could be suffering from an active toxo-plasmosis, with a considerable margin for increase. This is a high risk and the case studies clearly show how severely that illness can progress.*

11.5. Factors that promote a chronic active toxoplasmosis

The balance between our immune system and Toxoplasma gondii can shift to our disadvantage if the immune system is too weak to keep the parasite at bay (6). In humans who carry the parasite, severe health burdens, severe phases of exhaustion and possibly also very severe psychic strain could thus lead to a "reactivation", and a significant increase in a hitherto inactive toxoplasmosis. According to my experience this does not show at the same time as the burdening factor, but some weeks afterwards. I attribute this time lag to the parasites' need to "crank up" their metabolism. Other health burdens apart from those witnessed by me could also possibly favour the change from an inactive to a chronic active toxoplasmosis. Yet in many patients, the onset of the illness has happened years ago and physical ailments, which occurred prior to the creeping onset of symptoms can only rarely be remembered.

In the following cases, triggering factors could be determined:

In case 1 (from page 96), there were several factors that burdened the patient's health. These were a (treated) borreliosis, a chronic appendicitis with surgery, a vitamin D deficiency, and finally an acne inversa, i.e. an acne with severe purulent abscesses, which had to be operated on 3 times. About three months after the last surgery, the patient's condition worsened considerably. This was probably the time when an increased activity of Toxoplasma caused symptoms.

In case 6, (from page 108) symptoms occurred after 2 surgeries. At first, a part of the rectum had to be removed due to severe inflammation and two months later a follow-up surgery had to be performed in this region due to scarification.

The patient did not recover well from these surgeries and developed an active toxoplasmosis. I think that the first serious surgery had already posed the starting point for this development.

In case 7 (original work from page 34), a chronically purulent wound, which needed follow-up surgery four times had been persisting for four years after surgery. The patient developed increasing symptoms of an active toxoplasmosis about 2-3 months after the last surgery.

In case 17 (from page 130), the patient's symptoms of an active toxoplasmosis started about 3-4 weeks after several flu-like infections.

In cases 21 (from page 131) and 23 (original work from page 68), the symptoms of an active toxoplasmosis increased directly after pregnancy. **This results in a high risk for mistaking an active toxoplasmosis with a persisting post-natal depression. It is therefore sensible to ask such patients about the symptoms of an active toxoplasmosis also.**

In one young patient (case 19 from p.137), sweating and a loss of performance, the reason of which had been hidden at first, had been persisting 2 years prior to the beginning of the illness. Early in 2016 she suffered from mononucleosis (caused by the Epstein-Barr virus), from which she recovered at first. Some months after the mononucleosis, she suffered from several severe infections in short sequence. It became obvious that the symptoms of an active toxoplasmosis had been there before, but had increased considerably after the mononucleosis.

It is known that a Chronic Fatigue Syndrome (CFS) with abnormal tiredness, muscular pains and concentration disorders can occur after a mononucleosis (45, 87). It is conceivable that some of these cases of CFS can be attributed to a reactivation of Toxoplasma, and thus an effective way to treat these cases would be at hand.

11.6. Symptom intensities prior to and post therapy

In this chapter, I'd like to examine the severity and resulting reductions in symptoms reported by patients. Symptom intensities are presented in values from 0 to 10, and are reported first. The value for the rated intensity after therapy is shown in brackets after the intensity and then the symptom reduction as a percentage is given.

The intensities prior to therapy were generally a bit more pronounced in group A than in group B. Exceptions here are the symptoms listlessness, dizziness, oedema (i.e. swelling of feet and/or hands with water retention), and sleep disorders and anxieties, which exhibit a higher initial intensity in group B. A possible explanation could be that these symptoms were experienced as "atypical" and not "age-related" and thus considered stronger by the on-average younger patients of group B, which leads to higher rated intensity values.

The symptom reduction after therapy is generally somewhat better in group B than in group A, which I attribute to the shorter disease duration and the lower age in group B. There are observable differences between men and women with regards to the symptoms "irritability", "depressive moods", "anxieties" and "oedema". These gender-related differences still have to be assessed with caution, since there are only 6 men among the 27 cases.

The individual symptoms and their intensities before and after therapy in comparison in groups A and B will be discussed on the following pages.

Abnormal fatigue and a permanent profound tiredness affects all patients and is probably the earliest, most sensitive and unfortunately also most imprecise symptom of an active toxoplasmosis. Patients often have an intensive need for sleep, but sleep only reduces the tiredness for a short time. In 8 cases, sleep disorders were reported, which certainly contributed to the tiredness. The remaining 19 patients also suffered from an almost permanent fatigue, without having suffered from sleep disorders. I see the reason of this fatigue as **exhaustion caused by the disease.**

The symptom intensities of 8.8 (1.4) in group A and 8.6 (0.9) in group B amount to the highest values of all symptoms and are still comparatively high in group B despite the significantly shorter disease duration. This symptom probably reaches a considerable intensity at an early stage and is considered particularly burdensome independently of age. The symptom reductions of group A (85%) and group B (89%) show that this symptom can be improved very well by means of therapy.

Muscular pain and/or increased muscle cramping are also early symptoms in many cases, and affect all patients. They amount to an intensity of 8.2 (0.9) in group A and 6.5 (0.4) in group B. The pains can be located all over the body and may imitate fibromyalgia due to pressure-sensitive muscles (case 11 on p.114 and case 14 on p.120). The pains are often symmetrical and typically increase with light exertion. Most of the time, the upper leg muscles hurt from simply climbing stairs, or the patient feels very relieved to have "finally" managed to climb the stairs, since the muscles are often also weakened.

A shortness of breath often intensifies the problem (see p.173). In some cases, patients also report increased cramping or frequent involuntary contractions of single muscle bundles. In selected cases, as in case 25, the muscular pains can be of low intensity, and eventually cramping and/or weakness is more pronounced. An active toxoplasmosis should not simply be excluded if muscular problems are less noticeable. The symptom reduction is 90% in group A and 94% in group B.

Please note, if in some patients all symptoms of an active toxoplasmosis are in remission during therapy, but significant muscular symptoms remain, particular attention is needed, because: In some cases, toxoplasmosis can cause an illness which resembles the clinical picture of a rheumatoid inflammation of the muscle (a Polymyalgia rheumatica) to perfection.

This disease is explained on p. 66. Cases, in which a polymyalgia - imitating clinical picture has been triggered by toxoplasmosis have already been reported before and can be found in the scientific papers (7, 16, 63). In my patients this could be observed in case 27 (original paper), and I have subsequently seen several other patients with these symptoms after a chronic active toxoplasmosis. This is the reason why some scientists propose considering a toxoplasmosis as possible cause in diagnosing muscle inflammations (7, 63). After completion of a toxoplasmosis therapy it can be necessary in these cases to prescribe a low dosage of cortisone, similar to a "normal" Polymyalgia rheumatica.

Concentration disorders affect all patients excluding cases 10 and 27 and therefore 94% of group A and 90% of group B. Questions concerning word-finding disorders and disturbances of the short-term memory were particularly helpful when discussing the checklist. Some patients reported a significantly reduced learning ability as well as an impairment of professional activity. The symptoms were so burdening that some patients already voiced concerns about a possible dementia. The intensity of these symptoms has a tendency to increase with time. The intensities in group A were 7.8 (2.2) and 6.5 (1.3) in group B. The symptom reduction is slightly better in group B at 84% than in group A at 74%.

Increased sweating occurred in 14 patients (82%) of group A and in 7 patients (70%) of group B. The intensities in group A were 7.5 (1.3) and 8.8 (1.0) in group B. This is one of the few symptoms in which group B achieves a higher intensity than group A.

The patients reported about unusually intensive sweating with only light physical exertion and also frequently mentioned nocturnal sweating. This is a problem for women especially, since a relation with menopause is often initially considered. If sweating is only one symptom of a wider ranging symptomatic and improves during toxoplasmosis therapy, menopause obviously is *not* the decisive cause. The symptom reductions in group B (88%) and group A (84%) were almost the same.

Dyspnoea (shortness of breath) at light physical exertion has been reported by 11 patients (65%) of group A and 7 patients (70%) of group B. The initial intensities were in group A at 8.4 (1.8) and in group B at 7.4 (1.4), showing a good improvement with therapy. The impairment matched in one case (case 26) that of a 3rd grade heart insufficiency (up to NYHA III) and was often paired with a significantly increased pulse rate with only light physical exertion, as seen in cases 1, 5, 6 and 16. Several patients also reported an increased pulse while resting.

Some patients with dyspnoea also showed slight oedema, which also improved considerably during therapy (cases 1, 5, 8, 12, 14, 16 as well as 21 and 26). Many of the affected patients (in the cases 1, 2, 5, 6, 8 and 16 as well as 22, 24 and 26) had therefore undergone cardiological examination. Despite the oedema and the often significant dyspnoea, the findings were normal and no further explanation for these problems was found. In at least 2 cases the patient was advised to seek psychotherapy. It is possible that in these patients, dyspnoea had been caused by a toxoplasmosis-related heart muscle inflammation. A corresponding case is described in chapter 3; see p.25, Palo Alto 1994 (58). There are also clues in scientific literature with regards to an affliction of the lungs (11) and the diaphragm (53) due to an active toxoplasmosis.

It can therefore be assumed that in cases of active toxoplasmosis dyspnoea is caused by a combined affliction of the lungs, heart and diaphragm, and thus generally cannot be assigned to one single cause. The dyspnoea improved following toxoplasmosis therapy by 80% in group and by 82% in group B. **After the toxoplasmosis treatment, none of these patients suffered from dyspnoea gain.**

Listlessness was reported by 12 patients (70%) from group A and 5 patients (50%) from group B. It was mostly experienced as very burdening, since the complete daily routine and social life suffer permanently and significantly. This has been experienced as particularly tormenting by some patients, who had been very active previously, and who literally had to pull themselves together to get things done. Similar to the sweating, the intensities mentioned from group B were higher at an average of 8.8 (0.8) than those from group A at 8.1 (2.1).

The reduction of symptoms in group B of 90% as opposed to 76% in group A is noticeable. The younger age and the shorter disease duration are possibly positive factors here. It is pleasing that for most patents, this symptom improves significantly within the first 7 – 10 days of treatment and the patients often report about a very positive "boost of energy".

Addition in 10/2019: Some patients, who suffered from a chronic active toxoplasmosis to a very severe degree, which then resembles a **chronic fatigue syndrom (CFS)**, have pointed out, that "listlessness" does not describe their problem.
They are not precisely "listless", but permanently exhausted, they lack energy and have to gather all what is left to get simple tasks done – and after having fulfilled these, they are then tormented by a considerable worsening of their symptoms. I therefore modified the Checklist and added "exhaustion" to "listlessness", but I have to point out, that it is still a checklist for chronic active toxoplasmosis (CATOX), and discrimination between a CFS and CATOX can be very difficult.

On the following 4 pages symptoms will be discussed, which affect the psyche and here, differences in the fields of irritability, depressive moods and anxieties can be noticed between men and women. There are numerous studies dealing with neurological illness, severe impairment of the psyche and changes in behaviour that can be triggered by Toxoplasma (12, 22, 28, 29, 30, 31, 83, 91, 92, 93). Please note that the significance of this case study with reference to gender-related differences is limited, but still the differences seen are remarkable.

Symptoms comprise an increased risk for the occurrence of schizophrenia (22, 91, 92, 93), psychoses (92) or aggressive behaviour, also a doubling of the risk for accidents in cases where Toxoplasma antibodies have been detected (28). Explanations for that may point to the mentioned behavioural changes and the decreasing psychomotor resilience (39) due to Toxoplasma infections. It is scary that even an increase in the number of attempted suicides has been correlated with antibody detection in toxoplasmosis (22, 91).

It fits this bill that toxoplasmosis infected rats are known to lose all fear of cats. They literally seek them out in broad daylight, to be eaten in the end, a behaviour that is very advantageous for the spreading of Toxo-plasma, but not so good for the rat. The consequence is clear. When the host is "ripe" and contains many bradyzoite - cysts, it is simply more useful for the parasite when dead instead of alive, particularly if the death is caused by a cat. Death by car accident or suicide are thus somehow "inappropriate", but can be regarded as a somewhat macabre continuation of such behavioural disturbances in the present.

A detailed discussion of the neurological symptoms and the studies mentioned cannot be achieved within the scope of this book, however scientific literature which covers the topic in greater detail is available.

Significantly increased irritability could be found in 53% of group A and 40% of group B. The intensities were 8.6 (3.6) in group A and 7.0 (0.5) in group B. **The symptom reductions were 67% (A) and 90% (B).** Most patients were quite self-critical with regards to this symptom during anamnesis and mostly had the distinct feeling that their irritable, exuberant reactions in even moderately conflictive situations often had no comprehensible reason. They frequently reported they "exploded" for invalid reasons. They felt considerably unhappy with these reactions and some had familiar problems and/or problems at the workplace due to those behavioural changes. This symptom often improved surprisingly quickly with therapy.

Across both groups, 83% of men and 38% of women were affected, whereas the intensity mentioned by men was slightly higher at 8.2 (3.6) than the one at 8.0 (1.25) by women. *The symptom reduction of 56% in men was less than that in women (86%).*

> *To sum it up, an increased irritability due to Toxoplasma activity is more frequent in men than in women. Furthermore, they seem to be affected by the symptom after a shorter disease duration and more intensively than women, with a lesser decrease in symptoms.*

Depressive moods occurred in 41% of group A and 40% of group B. The intensities were at 8.0 (2.9) in group A and 7.5 (2.25) in group B. The average disease duration for those affected was 20.4 years for group A and thus about 10.4 years above the average of the combined group. In the 4 affected patients of group B, the average disease duration was about 10.8 years and thus 5 years above the combined average. This indicates depressive moods to be a typical symptom for longer disease durations. One patient had a symptom intensity of 7 (case 21) yet had only been suffering from an active toxoplasmosis for 3½ years, indicating this symptom may also occur significantly earlier. The symptom reductions of 65% (A) and 78% (B) led to a significant improvement of quality of life in the affected patients.

It is remarkable that only one in 6 men (17%) quoted a depressive disorder, but with an intensity of 10 (5) in contrast to 10 of 21 women (48%). The lone male (case 25) had a disease duration of 24 years, an age of 57 and a symptom reduction of 50%. In the 10 women who were affected by depressive moods, the average disease duration was 16.2 years and the average age was 49.9 years. In the women, the initial intensity was 7.6 (2.4) and the average reduction was 72%.

I would like to acknowledge a remarkable parallel. Based on recent research, Edward Bullmore, in his amazing book The Inflamed Mind, explains how cytokines (highly active messenger substances) can play a major role in the development of depression. There has been found proof, that tachyzoits as well as bradyzoits can induce certain cyto-kine responses in the brain (27) so it could be, that this is one of their ways to burden our health and to heavily influence the host's psyche.

Anxieties which occur uncontrolled in non-threatening situations are labelled as anxiety disorders. Six patients of group A (35%) as well as two patients (20%) of group B were suffering from this symptom. Those anxiety disorders are probably more likely to occur after longer disease durations, since the affected patients in group A had been suffering from the illness for 21 years on average and the patients in group B for 14 years. In case 9 a chronic active toxoplasmosis had only been existing for about 6 years, so this symptom may also occur earlier in the progression of the disease.

The affected patients considered their anxieties be inappropriate for the situation in most cases, similar to the increased irritability. Still they were unable to ignore their anxieties, resulting in a significant impairment of life-quality. Only one patient (case 25) is male. In other words, across groups, 7 of 21 women (33%) show this symptom, but only 1 in 6 men (17%).

The intensities were 8.3 (2.0) in group A and 8.5 (0.5) in group B. The symptom reduction of 76% (A) and 92% (B) point towards a good therapeutic efficacy. It is remarkable, that the improvement came usually within the first weeks of treatment.

The differences between men and women with regards to the psychic symptoms "irritability ", "depressive moods" and "anxiety" can be assumed to be that women are far more frequently affected by depressive moods and anxieties, and these symptoms tend to increase with longer disease duration. Many patients exhibit depressive moods as well as anxieties, so there are also overlaps.

The symptom "irritability" however is more frequent in men, occurring slightly earlier, connected to a slightly higher intensity and a worse symptom reduction. This leads to the impression that the more frequently increased irritability in men is in some respect the male counterpart to the relatively more frequent depressive moods and increased anxieties in women.

Visual disturbances   occurred in 9 patients of group A (53%) and 3 patients (30%) of group B. These patients all reported about an intermittent visual disorder, which was mostly described as "blurry" sight, in part caused by longer reading or exhaustion. The average intensities were not really high at 6.6 (4.3) in group A and 4.0 (0.67) in group B, but were experienced at the time as being very disturbing, some of these patients also described burning sensations of the eyes.

Almost all affected patients had been examined ophthalmologically before, without a cause for their disturbed sight or burning sensations being found. In several cases patients had already purchased new corrective glasses, without their sight being improved. The visual disturbances improved in only 4 of 9 patients in group A.   In these patients the intensities were 5.25 (0.25), a symptom reduction of 96%.

An improvement of the visual disorder thus only occurred in a minority of the affected patients from group A, yet the result in these patients was very good. Astonishingly, the visual disorder improved very well in *all* affected patients from Group B, with an average symptom reduction of 80%.   Burning sensations of the eyes, if present, vanished completely.

If the ophthalmological findings are inconspicuous, as it is the case in all of the presented cases, the most plausible explanation for that type of visual disorder in connection with a chronic active toxoplasmosis is a processing disorder of the optical image in the sight centre of the brain. This is most easily visualised as a "concentration disorder" in the sight centre of the brain.

In English-speaking countries such a visual disorder is described as "cortical visual impairment", which typically entails a "blurred vision". Infections of the so-called TORCH group, of which toxoplasmosis is a part, are considered responsible. I couldn't find a study which has investigated this kind of visual disturbance in connection with a *chronic active toxoplasmosis, so* this is only a possible explanation, but a very plausible one.

Unfocussed vertigo in combination with insecurity of gait occurred in 7 patients (41%) of group A and 3 patients (30%) of group B. The intensities in Group A were 6.4 (1.4) and 7.0 (0.0) in group B. The organ of equilibrium has been examined in all these patients, but no disturbances could be found. The patients typically reported about intermittent vertigo and the descriptions show some similarity to the visual disorders in that respect. Mostly, a vertigo without directional preference and an increased undirected staggering was described.

The maintenance of equilibrium is a highly complex joint accomplishment of the equilibrium organ inside the inner ear, the cerebellum and depth perception.

If only one part of this cooperation is even slightly disturbed, for example due to an active toxoplasmosis, vertigo can be the result. It has already been proved that gait insecurity can be caused by Toxoplasma activity inside the cerebellum (37). The improvement of 70% (A) and 100% (B) show that this complex of symptoms can be treated well.

Oedema, i.e. water retention in the hands and / or feet occurred in 6 patients (35%) of group A and 3 patients (30%) of group B. In group A the intensities were 6.6 (2.0) and in group B 7.6 (0.0). In the hands these fluid retentions often led to tensions which impaired fist closure. All patients who showed such swellings also suffered from dyspnoea, which can be assumed to have been partially caused by a heart insufficiency (56), impaired function of the lungs (11) as well as a possible involvement of the diaphragm (53). All in all, the symptom reductions of 65% (A) and 100% (B) point towards an effective therapy of water retention. Except for patient 25, all affected persons were female.

I tend to consider that this is a swelling of the connective tissue most of the time, which is caused by an activity of Toxoplasma in the connective tissue. In this respect most interesting are the cases 5 (p. 102) and 12 (p. 117). In these patients, lipoedema had already been diagnosed. This is a mixture of water and fat deposits in the connective tissue, which is haunting for women due to their softer connective tissue and which responds poorly to usual therapy. Astonishingly, these symptoms improved very well under toxoplasmosis therapy in these women, from 7 to 0 (case 5) and from 10 to 0 (case 12).

Morning stiffness   occurred in 5 patients (29%) of group A and 3 patients (30%) of group B. The symptom intensities were 8.0 (0.6) in group A and 8.0 (0.0) in group B. **The symptom reduction was 95% in group A and 100% in group B.** Half of the affected patients (cases 5, 8, 14 and 27) had been suspected to suffer from a rheumatoid disease previously (seronegative rheumatism, rheumatoid monoarthritis), however, the prescribed treatments had little effect. The symptoms only improved due to toxoplasmosis therapy. A certain resemblance, and therefore potential danger of confusion, between active toxoplasmosis and an active rheumatoid disease in terms of morning stiffness and joint pains must be noted.

Sleep disorders occurred in 5 patients (29%) of group A and 3 patients (30%) of group B. These patients especially reported about sleep maintenance insomnia with frequent and long-lasting nocturnal insomnia and impaired ability to fall asleep again. The symptom intensities were at 7.8 (2.2) in group A and at 8.0 (0.0) in group B. The average symptom reduction was 72% in group A and 100% in group B.

....

The symptoms **"insecure gait/impaired coordination"**, **"headaches"**, and **"joint aches"** which are part of the "Checklist toxoplasmosis" are missing here for a simple reason.

Around 2016/2017, when these cases were documented, I wasn't aware that these symptoms can be caused by a chronic active toxoplasmosis, so I didn't ask for these symptoms systematically, and a question not asked is an answer not given. We do need the right questions.

I always asked for swollen lymph nodes and searched for them, but I seldom found them. The most probable reason is that the sources that name "swollen lymph nodes" as a typical symptom of toxoplasmosis, deal with *acute courses of this disease*, which in many aspects shows differences to *chronic active toxoplasmosis*. Nevertheless, "swollen lymph nodes" is a part of the updated version of the checklist, but this symptom still belongs with those with little frequency and thus has little relevance in diagnosing chronic active toxoplasmosis.

11.7 Overview of average results

The overview of the average results on the following pages 186 / 187 should be understood as follows. The tables show symptoms, followed by the percent of the group showing the symptom, followed by the rating scale with a red X showing the average rating. The rating scale is repeated to show values after treatment, again with a red X showing the average rating, followed by the calculated reduction as a percent of the original rating "score".

As an example, all patients in   group A suffered from an increased fatigue, which yields a symptom frequency of 100%. The intensity of this symptom was an average of 9 in the beginning and after conclusion of the treatment it was slightly above 1. The average symptom reduction for this symptom is 85%.

Personal remark:

I am well aware that the group of 27 patients, on which the statistics are based, is too small to be understood as a scientific proof. Please keep in mind that the aim of the original work was never to present a "final" proof. This normally requires a full-sized medical department. The book at hand is still based on personal experience and documentation and an unknown amount of labour to research the background and to finally write this book.

I unfortunately failed in motivating "big medicine" to step in and to perform a full scientific study. Most of "them" are just not interested. This is why I wrote this book. It is mainly for those who are suffering from this disease. I just cannot wait until someday a sort of medical "white knight" appears and solves this problem for me, because there are seriously ill people who need help soon, not in 10 or 15 years.

So, this is my way to spread the news. This disease is by no means "under control", the wind blows entirely the other direction. We do have the means to deal with this disease, probably even heal it in the majority of cases. The question is when we will start to use all our scientific and medical power to do so.

There are excellent researchers and medical departments out there, but I am trying to start the "upload" of an idea to the medical machine, and this is quite an undertaking, because the machine is designed to work "downwards".

The general idea is that new ideas and wisdom are worked out at universities, passed down to hospitals, then passed down to doctors in their practises and in turn passed down to patients. As you might have noticed, I don't believe in "passing down". I believe in "networking". I do so every day in my practice, and some of the improvements in my daily work can be traced back to amazing questions and sometimes surprisingly well-informed patients. We need to listen to them carefully because it pays off.

Right now, I am looking back on well over 150 treated "toxoplasmosis cases", but as long as I am still a committed full time working general practitioner, it just far exceeds my personal ability to deal with this amount of data and to include it in this book. It is inevitable that we do need a big study that would focus on chronic active toxoplasmosis, because only such a study could be a real game changer for the good of our patients.

Overview of average results - group A, 17 patients

Age: 56 years **Duration** **10 years**

Toxoplasma **IgG** **75 U/ml** **IgM** **< 3 AU/ml**

	In the beginning	**After 4 weeks**
Symptom frequency%		**Symptom reduction %**

Symptom	Freq%	In the beginning	After 4 weeks	Reduction %
Fatigue	**100%**	0 1 2 3 4 5 6 7 8 X 10	0 1X 2 3 4 5 6	**85%**
Muscular pain	**100%**	0 1 2 3 4 5 6 7 X 9 10	0 X 2 3 4 5 6	**90%**
Concentration - Disorder	**94%**	0 1 2 3 4 5 6 7 X 9 10	0 1 X 3 4 5 6	**75%**
Sweating	**82%**	0 1 2 3 4 5 6 7X8 9 10	0 1 X 3 4 5 6	**84%**
Dyspnea	**65%**	0 1 2 3 4 5 6 7 8X9 10	0 1 X 3 4 5 6	**80%**
Listlessness	**70%**	0 1 2 3 4 5 6 7X 9 10	0 1 X 3 4 5 6	**76%**
Irritability	**70%**	0 1 2 3 4 5 6 7 8X 9 10	0 1 2 X 4 5 6	**70%**
Visual disturbance	**53%**	0 1 2 3 4 5 6X7 8 9 10	0 1 2 3 X 5 6	**42%**
Dizziness	**41%**	0 1 2 3 4 5 6X 7 8 9 10	0 1X 2 3 4 5 6	**74%**
Depressive moods	**41%**	0 1 2 3 4 5 6 7X 9 10	0 1 2 X 4 5 6	**65%**
Anxieties	**35%**	0 1 2 3 4 5 6 7 8X9 10	0 1 X 3 4 5 6	**76%**
Morning stiffness	**29%**	0 1 2 3 4 5 6 7X9 10	0X1 2 3 4 5 6	**95%**
Oedema	**35%**	0 1 2 3 4 5 6X7 8 9 10	0 1 X 3 4 5 6	**65%**
Sleeping disorder	**29%**	0 1 2 3 4 5 6 7 X9 10	0 1 X 3 4 5 6	**72%**
Pressure in upper abdomen	**20%**	0 1 2 3 4 5 6 7 8 X 10	0 1X2 3 4 5 6	**81%**

Overview of average results - group B, 10 patients

Age: 43 years   **Duration**   **6 years**

Toxoplasma   **IgG**   **< 3 U/ml**   **IgM**   **< 3 AU/ml**

In the beginning   **After 4 weeks**

Symptom frequency%   **Symptom reduction %**

Symptom	Freq.	In the beginning	After 4 weeks	Reduction
Fatigue	100%	0 1 2 3 4 5 6 7 8X9 10	0X 2 3 4 5 6	89%
Muscular pain	100%	0 1 2 3 4 5 6X7 8 9 10	0X1 2 3 4 5 6	94%
Concentration - Disorder	90%	0 1 2 3 4 5 6X7 8 9 10	0 1X2 3 4 5 6	75%
Sweating	70%	0 1 2 3 4 5 6 7 8 X 10	0 X 2 3 4 5 6	88%
Dyspnea	70%	0 1 2 3 4 5 6 7X8 9 10	0 1X2 3 4 5 6	82%
Listlessness	50%	0 1 2 3 4 5 6 7 8 X10	0 X 2 3 4 5 6	90%
Irritability	40%	0 1 2 3 4 5 6 7X8 9 10	0X1 2 3 4 5 6	60%
Visual disturbance	30%	0 1 2 3 X 5 6 7 8 9 10	0X1 2 3 4 5 6	80%
Dizziness	30%	0 1 2 3 4 5 6 X 8 9 10	X 1 2 3 4 5 6	100%
Depressive moods	40%	0 1 2 3 4 5 6 7X8 9 10	0 1 X 3 4 5 6	78%
Anxieties	20%	0 1 2 3 4 5 6 7 8X9 10	0X1 2 3 4 5 6	92%
Morning stiffness	30%	0 1 2 3 4 5 6 7 X 9 10	X 1 2 3 4 5 6	100%
Oedema	30%	0 1 2 3 4 5 6 7X8 9 10	X 1 2 3 4 5 6	100%
Sleeping disorder	30%	0 1 2 3 4 5 6 7X8 9 10	0 1X3 4 5 6	72%
Pressure in upper abdomen	17%	0 1 2 3 4 5 6 7 8X 10	0 1 2 3 X 5 6	65%

12.   Therapy of an active toxoplasmosis

An important note beforehand: patients with immune deficiencies or undergoing an immune-suppressive/immune-modulating therapy, for example following organ transplants, during cancer treatment or under certain antirheumatic drugs have a high risk, and should therefore be observed very closely or even better be treated in hospital. In these patients, the prescription of pyrimethamine (Daraprim) or sulfadiazine must only be undertaken with utmost care.

12.1. Start of therapy

Since I could not be sure at the beginning of this whole series of treatments if patients were suffering from an active toxoplasmosis in all cases because of contradictory laboratory findings, I started to look for a way to start treatment without necessarily having to prescribe a combination therapy at once. By 1993, the effectiveness of a therapy with clindamycin alone had been proven (9). clindamycin has been produced since 1967 and is mostly used in the treatment of infections of the soft tissue, bones and ear.

In cases of pronounced symptoms or a very long disease duration it is advisable to prescribe not more than 3 x 300mg clindamycin at first, since in some cases an initial worsening of symptoms in the first 3 – 4 days with a temporary increase in fatigue and muscular pains may occur. In all other cases, a dosage of 2 x 600mg for a duration of 7 – 10 days has proven its worth. The patients often describe noticeable improvements already within the first week of treatment, which generally clearly shows on the checklist.

The first week's improvements are mostly related to a decrease in muscular pains and fatigue. Often irritability and aggression are also decreased, if they existed at all. The concentration disorders, visual disturbances and sweating generally only decrease slightly in the beginning and start to improve significantly after 2-3 weeks of therapy. In some cases, with a shorter disease duration and moderately pronounced symptoms, a therapy with clindamycin alone for four weeks can sometimes yield good or very good improvements and a combination therapy may then be foregone.

Clindamycine unfortunately shares a disadvantage of many other antibiotics, as it also kills beneficial intestinal microorganisms, and can thereby trigger bouts of diarrhoea. In more severe cases an antibiotics-related inflammation of the gut, due to the elimination of useful beneficial intestinal microorganisms may occur. This risk can be reduced by parallel ingestion of a *saccharomyces boulardii* preparation twice daily (sold under the brand names "Perenterol" or "Yomogi"). Should diarrhoea occur, increased care is to be taken and the practitioner has to be consulted. In case of doubt, the clindamycin administration has to be stopped.

It is hard to predict the reliability of such a clindamycin trial. This could only be done precisely by means of a study. According to my experience, an "effective rate" of approximately 70 % can be achieved, if one runs an effective differential diagnosis and uses the checklist consistently. In most cases of an effective clindamycin therapy, a combination therapy is significantly more effective.

In cases of an ineffective clindamycin therapy, a combination therapy will be of no use, most of the times. (see original work p.15). Possible reasons for the missing efficacy in some cases will be discussed on p. 216. In case of an intolerance to clindamycin, I use Spiramycine (Rovamycine) 1.5 mio 4x1 up to 3x2 as initial medication (see also p. 184). I cannot confidently answer if that would be as effective as clindamycin for the continuation of the therapy in a larger group of patients. With good efficacy after a 7–10-day therapy with Rovamicine, I generally only prescribe this medication for the remaining time of treatment, since it is effective as a single medication in most cases.

> *It has been seen in the therapy of almost all cases in which Clinda-mycin was effective within the first 7-10 days, that a very good result with the combination therapy followed.*

12.2. Combination therapies

A combination therapy is prescribed for about 3-4 weeks, depending on the effectiveness, and, in very severe cases, up to 10 weeks. It should only be stopped when all symptoms of an active toxoplasmosis have been eliminated almost completely. During this therapy, kidney and liver values, blood count and folic acid level should be monitored. A combination of 3 drugs is usually employed.

The two drugs described on the next page are part of each combination of 3 drugs. Several different antibiotics that will be described in detail can be used as the third partner in these combinations of three drugs.

Pyrimethamine

(Brand-name Daraprim) is used in a dosage of 25mg 2x1 tablet per day. The drug was discovered in 1952 and it is approved as a treatment against toxoplasmosis in combination with certain antibiotics. Pyrimethamine suppresses an enzyme which is essential for the supply of the vital folic acid. The resulting deficiency in folic acid damages Toxoplasma significantly. **Beware however, as it is vitally important to ingest folinic acid (calcium folinate) during the administration of this drug!!**

This is necessary because otherwise the human organism would suffer from a folacin impoverishment at the same time, and this could cause life-threatening side-effects. Toxoplasma cannot utilise folinic acid, so that only they suffer from a folacin impoverishment. This leads us to the next drug.

Calcium folinate

capsules with 15mg and tablets with 6.35mg are available. The ingestion of 1 capsule of calcium folinate 15mg every second day usually leads to a slight increase of the folic acid level under Daraprim therapy. One tablet with 6.35mg can be ingested daily as an alternative. At a price of about 22 Euros (about 25$US) for 50 tablets, this is an economic alternative. The folic acid level must be monitored, as I have noted.

Beware: cheaper folic acid may under no circumstance be used as a substitute. It would be inefficient in this case and the resulting folacin impoverishment would be dangerous !! (55)

Sulfadiazine 500mg 4x1 up to 4x2 tablets

per day is an antibiotic from the group of sulphonamides and may therefore not be used in patients with sulphonamide allergies. The effectiveness derives from a suppression of the production of folic acid, so it supplements the effectiveness of pyrimethamine (Daraprim) substantially. Sulfadiazine is only approved as a treatment against toxoplasmosis in combination with pyrimethamine. Unfortunately, side-effects such as nausea and headaches are frequent, which is why I usually prescribe only 4 tablets, and in some cases even 3 tablets per day. If side-effects or a loss of therapeutic effectiveness can be observed, a different antibiotic has to be prescribed instead of sulfadiazine, which then has to be combined with Daraprim and calcium folinate.

Clindamycine 3x300mg or 2x600mg

Its effectivity is almost equivalent to sulfadiazine (40). I sometimes directly prescribe it as combination partner first, if it proves a good effectiveness in the 7-10 days initial phase without causing side-effects. For side effects see p.189. In cases in which clindamycin has proved to be very effective and has shown a good tolerability at the initial stage, a combination therapy can sometimes be foregone. Headaches, which frequently occur under Sulfadiazine, rarely occur under clindamycin.

Cotrimoxazole 960mg 2x1

is another alternative. It also contains a sulphonamide and belongs to the same group as Sulfadiazine. It is a combination drug of sulfamethoxazole and trimethoprim. Both substances inhibit the synthesis of tetrahydrofolic acid and thus function similarly to sulfadiazine. Thus, Cotrimoxazole is not the first choice as second-line medication, if a combination therapy with Sulfadiazine does not show sufficient effectiveness. There is less risk for antibiotics-induced diarrhoea than under clindamycin

Spiramycine 1.5mio 4x1 up to 3x2

can be obtained under the brand-name "Rovamycine", belongs to the group of the makrolides and can be combined with pyrimethamine and calcium folinate, but it is also effective as a monotherapy. This makes it interesting especially for patients who cannot tolerate a combination therapy. I have also used it as an initial medication in cases of a clindamycine intolerance.

According to body weight, 4x1 up to 3x2 tablets of 1.5 million units are prescribed and use is prolonged in case of high effectiveness. From my point of view, this mostly shows a slightly increased effectiveness compared to clindamycine alone, but a slightly decreased effectiveness in combination therapy. A combination of Rovamycine, Daraprim and calcium folinate is possible but, according to my experience, it is not always tolerated well.

These are the tried and tested therapies, which are available in our daily practice and which help us to achieve our goal, which is the almost complete reduction of toxoplasmosis symptoms. More intensive progressions of the disease may require higher dosages, potentially other drug combinations and a longer duration of therapy (40, 41). One should also consider admittance to a hospital in such severe cases.

Medication weakens Toxoplasma gondii significantly and takes the pressure off our immune system, so that it can regain the upper hand again. This effect remains intact even months after the therapy, nevertheless experience has shown that Toxoplasma will recover sooner or later and will increase its activity again.

This is called a "relapse" (see also 12.5 from p.202). Every affected patient should be informed about this since it is sensible to start therapy again quickly in case of the reoccurrence of toxoplasmosis symptoms, before Toxoplasma can again weaken the immune system too much. Relapses can usually be treated very well. I generally again prescribe the last successful medication. Relapses become less intensive with every treatment and the symptom free intervals get longer over time.

In the long run, there might be medication available, which will be more effective against Toxoplasma in tissue cysts (21, 57), and only then we can hope that there won't be any more relapses after a successful therapy.

It is imperative to monitor the patient in the course of therapy in frequent consultations and I found 10-day intervals to be appropriate. This serves to find out about potential side-effects or losses of effectiveness, and to adjust or change the therapy accordingly. This is needed in about 30% of all cases.

In specific cases a "revolving" therapy in intervals of 5 days has to be considered and by doing so the adaption of Toxoplasma to the therapy can be effectively avoided. This will be discussed in 12.4. on pages 200 and 201 as "revolving therapy concept".

....

12.3. Alternative therapies

In case of allergies to antibiotics or side-effects, one possibly has to switch to alternative therapies. All drugs mentioned here can be used in the treatment of toxoplasmosis, but these would be "off label"-prescriptions.

The drugs are, in theory, not meant to be used for treatment of an active toxoplasmosis, since their effectiveness against Toxoplasma had not been proved at the time of licensing. This sounds unusual, but it may certainly happen in the practitioner's work, since sometimes further valuable therapeutic effects of the medication are only registered years after licensing. An additional licensing is very expensive and arduous, which is why the pharmaceutical companies often refrain from it and a prescription of the drug in this new range of application will then automatically be described as an "off label" prescription.

If an "off label" prescription is not avoidable, statutory health insurances might not cover these private prescriptions. Insurance companies would probably also argue that a person with a negative IgM cannot suffer from an active toxoplasmosis, so this claim will be hard to refute.

Clarithromycin 500mg 2x1 up to 2x2

This is a conventional antibiotic and is used in the daily practice for the treatment of infections of the respiratory system. Similar to Spiramycine (brand-name Rovamycine), it belongs to the group "macrolides" and is therefore very similar in its effect. It has been proven to be a useful alternative partner for a triple therapy together with Daraprim and calcium folinate (40).

Azithromycin 500-600mg 1x1

This is also a macrolide and it can be used as a combination partner for pyrimethamine and calcium folinate, just like Clarithromycin (40). It is effectively used in the therapy of borreliosis, with 500-600mg once a day for 4 days, then the therapy is stopped for 3 days so the substance does not accumulate excessively in the cells due to its slow degradation. According to information gathered in a talk with Dr. Hopf-Seidel, who has a years-long professional experience treating borreliosis, Azithromycin is tolerated well if taken intermittently for even a longer time.

Atovaquone 200mg 1x1

is a malaria remedy and can be used for the treatment of toxoplasmosis in combination with Daraprim and calcium folinate (40). As already mentioned at the beginning of this book, the pathogens of malaria and Toxoplasma gondii are closely related, so the effectiveness of Atovaquone against both pathogens comes as no surprise.

In the treatment of malaria, up to 4 tablets of Atovaquone are to be taken initially. If it is the first drug prescribed, I would recommend no more than two tablets per day for the first three days to check tolerance, and then switching to 1x1 per day. Since the drug has a longer half-life of 2-3 days, the dosage has to be reduced to, for example, one tablet every 2-3 days in the course of the treatment. This is done with a continuing Daraprim and calcium folinate intake. It has to be pointed out in favour of the drug that it is inefficient against bacteria so an impairment of the intestinal flora is not expected.

Colchicine up to 2 mg per day

Colchicine is only available by prescription. It is the poison of the meadow saffron, one of the oldest medical substances for the treatment of gout, and it is the only plant-based alternative known to me. It is effective against Toxoplasma, which was discovered in 1996 (1). The traditionally high doses for treating a gout flare (up to 8 mg per day) are no longer appropriate, as it has been found, that a lower dose (up to 2 mg per day) is effective, while delivering fewer side effects.

In my personal experience, treating chronic acitve toxoplasmosis with 1.5 mg colchicine per day works effectively, but the effect is weaker than an antibiotic / Daraprim / calcium folinate combination – and thus colchicine is inappropriate for more severe progressions of an chronic active toxoplasmosis.

I don't recommend a higher dosage, and certainly **no combination with other antibiotics or drugs**, because the metabolization of colchicine might be impaired by other drugs that are metabolized via the same biochemical pathway. This could result in stronger side effects. The instruction leaflet included with the prescription should be examined carefully. In elderly patients or patients with renal or hepatical impairment, a reduced dose should be considered.

Prescribing colchicine for the treatment of chronic active toxoplasmosi is an "off-label" prescription, and it should only be considered as a therapeutic alternative in selected cases if a conventional therapy can not be taken due to several intolerances.

Beware: The meadow saffron is a poisonous plant and the substance has to be handled and taken with care, and should only be prescribed by a doctor. I also strongly advise following the instruction leaflet and to carry out regular checks of the blood values, with frequent checks of the liver and kidney values to prevent side-effects.

12.4. The revolving therapy concept

After I had begun to integrate toxoplasmosis treatments in my daily work, I soon had to face the first difficulties in treating chronic active toxoplasmosis. In some cases (approximately 20-30%), the initial clindamycin trial was usually a success, but lost its effectiveness after approximately a week, as could happen with the alternatives as well.

It took some time until I realised that this loss of efficacy never set in before the 6th day of treatment and in some cases, it occurred only after 10 days of treatment. It is known that our therapies are not able to kill Toxoplasma, so in some cases the parasites seem to be able to adapt to the medication. A possible solution would be to combine more antibiotics, but this might also significantly increase the side effects. I therefore decided for a "revolving concept", which changes the combinations regularly after 5 days, *before* toxoplasma have fully adapted and it has been proven to be highly useful in my daily work. It is performed as follows:

- Pyrimethamine 25 mg 2 x 1 and Calcium folinate 6.35 mg 1 x 1 is taken continuously. It seems, that Toxoplasma can't avoid the resulting folic acid deprivation. For 5 days an antibiotic is added, for example

- Sulfadiazine 500 mg 4 x 1, changed after 5 days to, for example

- Clindamycin 600 mg 2 x 1, changed after 5 days to, for example,

- Clarithromycin 500 mg 2 x 1, and after 5 days this has also changed.

At that point the first antibiotic usually again shows a good result, as will be the case with the other antibiotics. They are then prescribed in the same order, until the symptoms disappear.

So, however Toxoplasma adapt, fortunately their metabolism seems to allow only adaptation to one combination of drugs at a time. The single combinations have to be adjusted for each patient, depending on the efficacy and possible side effects. Another example for such a therapy concept could be this:

- Pyrimethamine 25 mg 2 x 1 and Calciumfolinate 6,35 mg 1 x 1 is taken continuously. An antiobiotic is added, for example

- Clindamycine 600 mg 2 x 1, changed after 5 days to, for example,

- Cotrimoxazol 960 mg 2 x 1, changed after 5 days to, for example,

- Spiramycine 1,5mio 4x1 up to 3x2. As this drug is effective against Toxoplasma alone; without Daraprim and Calciumfolinate, these two drugs can be discontinued while taking Spiramycin.

After 5 days the therapy is continued with a combination of Pyrimethamine, Calciumfolinate and Clindamycine, and so on, until the symptoms have nearly completely subsided. A third revolving combination was prescribed in two LTT-positive cases (see pp. 214 - 220)

Therapy needs to be performed for at least 4 weeks , with a following relapse prophylaxis (see page 204). In the long run, there will be need for research, that focuses on the presumed ability of toxoplasma to adjust their metabolism, as it can impair the effiacy of treatments.

12.5. Relapses (recurrences) are possible – but well treatable

Toxoplasma are very resilient and at the moment, eradication is beyond our scope and thus relapses (recurrences) are possible. The risk of a relapse possibly increases due to health-related factors, such as severe viral infections, unusually high IgG values, long progressions of the disease or a very short duration of treatment.

In my patients, 5 relapses occurred by the end of January 2017, and the end of treatment had not been that long ago in some cases. In my daily practice I experienced a rising number of relapses if the toxoplasmosis treatment has been completed for some time, but I cannot quote precise figures. It is still encouraging that all **patients who suffered from a relapse have responded very well to a renewed treatment.** The time in which patients were free from symptoms varied considerably between 2 weeks (case 25) and 16 months (case 27); the average time was about 4 ½ months. To my experience, the relapses get weaker with every treatment.

Case 5 is the patient with the longest disease duration (50 years) and a high disease intensity, and she suffered from a relapse after only 3 weeks. The renewed combination therapy was very effective.   The patient took a combination therapy once a week for another 2 months to prevent another relapse.

In case 17 the disease had been persisting for only 7 months, yet the high Toxoplasma IgG (above 400 IU/ml, above measuring range) pointed towards a very strong tachyzoite activity. The relapse occurred only 6 weeks after the end of therapy. Such a constellation seems to trigger an increased risk for relapses.

In case 23 no factor apart from the long disease duration of 15 years could be determined that caused a relapse after 9 months.

In case 25 with a disease duration of 24 years, the relapse after 2 weeks was facilitated by the fact that the treatment had been abandoned after only 12 days due to side-effects.

In case 27 with a relapse after 16 months, an interaction with a muscle inflammation possible favoured the relapse. This is dealt with in greater detail in the case study and the according comment (see pp. 79-82).

In the months following the completion of the first case collection more relapses occurred, all of which could be dealt with effectively. The latest development concerning relapses (in cases 1, 7 and 17) is described on page 133. The Toxoplasma LTT of these patients showed positive results confirming the diagnosis. More accurate figures could be compiled by a study, ideally with a larger number of patients and a longer follow-up period. According to my experience, the relapses get weaker over time if they are treated in a timely way, so that in the long term most patients will eventually become completely free from symptoms.

> *All patients should be informed about the possibility of such a relapse and should see a doctor whenever a renewed Toxoplasma activity occurs. There is absolutely no advantage in "enduring" such a relapse for a longer time. The therapy of the relapses has been unanimously described by all patients as being faster and more effective than the first combination therapy.*

12.6. Prophylaxis of relapses

Relapses (recurrences) cannot be fully avoided, because that would require a complete eradication of Toxoplasma and that is unfortunately not yet possible. But it is also doubtful if that would be necessary in any case, since our immune system should be able to keep Toxoplasma under control to the degree that they become asymptomatic. There are no guidelines for the prevention of recurrences, only personal experiences. The following procedures have proven to be effective:

1. In the first block of treatment the medication needs to be taken continuously every day until the patient is free from symptoms; this usually takes between 4 and 6 weeks. In some cases a revolving therapy has to be applied (see p. 200 and 201) .

2. For a period of one month, the last successful combination therapy is taken on two treatment days per week (e.g. Wednesday and Sunday).

3. For a period of a second month, the last successful combination therapy is taken once per week.

It is sometimes sensible to vary this schedule slightly in patients with very severe or very lengthy progressions of the disease. In the first month of relapse prevention, treatment would be taken on 3 days per week and in the second month on 2 days per week. This therapeutic scheme is worth all the effort necessary to determine the course of action. In my experience, a relapse happens after that type of prophylaxis much later or not at all.

13. Outpatients

Some patients with an active toxoplasmosis have been transferred to our surgery for a toxoplasmosis treatment. The case of a 56-year old patient who had been suffering from an active toxoplasmosis for about 15 years is one of them. I will present my report to my colleague in slightly changed form here. The explanations set in italics have been added for better understanding. The checklist toxoplasmosis on p.208 shows the results of the first consultation on 19th September 2017 and the last consultation on 14th December 2017.

Dear colleague, thank you for the transferral of your patient Ms X

Anamnesis:

Since age 20 palpitations *(increased beating of the heart)* with initially normal physical resilience. For about 10 years recurring pains and inflammations in the mid foot have been persisting, as well as frequent severe bouts of sweating. Persisting absolute arrhythmia for about 7 years *(a frequent disturbance of the cardiac rhythm)*, unclear sleep-through disorders and an almost permanent fatigue for 5 years, 3 years ago an unclear visual disorder with frequent "blurry sight" was added. For one year at least, unusually severe muscular pains persist, which are felt after light physical exertion, but which can also occur at rest; additional unclear joint pains in the elbow and finger joints; moderate concentration disorders.

The patient explained that she had become very slow, her arms and legs felt "like lead". During initial contact in the surgery, her gait indeed appeared to be significantly slowed, the patient literally dragged herself along.

The presented laboratory values showed no conspicuous findings, apart from an increased sedimentation at 41/70mm and a positive Toxoplasma IgG; no detection of a folic acid deficiency.

11/2017 Toxoplasma check: several toxoplasmosis symptoms with a high score – thus a very high risk for an active toxoplasmosis persists. Toxoplasma IgG positive at 30 IU/ml, IgM negative. A slow progression of the symptoms for 15 years, reported by the patient, can be seen as typical.

Therapy: Under 3x300mg clindamycin from 20th September 2017 an initial worsening within the first days of treatment occurred. Ms X. felt increased muscular pains, which reduced again during the antibiotic therapy, a feeling of weight over the whole body, as well as a slight increase in concentration- and visual disorders. At the same time, exertional dyspnoea (*being short of breath*), morning stiffness as well as oedemas (*water retention*) improved. After 7 days, a reduction of dosage to 2x150mg clindamycin was arranged; symptoms still improved with a slightly better tolerance of the medication, so that the dosage could again be increased to 3x300 mg clindamycin. From 6th October 2017, Daraprim 2x25mg and calcium folinate 15mg 1x1   every second day could be prescribed. This medication was continued with steady improvement of the symptoms for 6 weeks; from the 26th November 2017, a reduction to 2 days of treatment per week as relapse prevention was prescribed, which was to be continued until the end of January 2018. A relapse is still possible despite prophylaxis; in that case, the combination therapy should be prescribed again at short notice.

With kind collegial regards, Dr. med. U. Auf der Straße

Checklist Toxoplasmosis

Mr/Mrs. ......X...

Age:..56...years	Duration.....15.....years	Intervalls yes / **no**
Toxoplasma	IgG 30.IU/ml	IgM................0..AU/ml
	Date: 19.9.2017	Date: 14.12.2017

Treatment:	Clindamycin 3 x 300 mg...	Clindamycini/ Daraprim ......Calciumfolinat...........
Fatigue	0 1 2 3 4 5 6 **X** 8 9 10	**X** 1 2 3 4 5 6 7 8 9 10
Muscular pains	0 1 2 3 4 5 6 7 **X** 9 10	**X** 1 2 3 4 5 6 7 8 9 10
Concentration disorders	0 1 2 3 4 5 **X** 7 8 9 10	0 1 **X** 3 4 5 6 7 8 9 10
Sweating	0 1 2 3 4 5 6 7 8 **X** 10	0 **X** 2 3 4 5 6 7 8 9 10
Dispnoea	0 1 2 3 4 5 6 **X** 8 9 10	**X** 1 2 3 4 5 6 7 8 9 10
Listlessness	0 1 2 3 4 5 6 7 **X** 9 10	0 **X** 2 3 4 5 6 7 8 9 10
Irritability	0 1 2 3 4 **X** 6 7 8 9 10	0 1 **X** 3 4 5 6 7 8 9 10
Visual disturbance	0 1 2 3 4 5 **X** 7 8 9 10	**X** 1 2 3 4 5 6 7 8 9 10
Dizziness	0 1 2 3 4 5 6 **X** 8 9 10	**X** 1 2 3 4 5 6 7 8 9 10
Depressive moods	0 1 **X** 3 4 5 6 7 8 9 10	0 **X** 2 3 4 5 6 7 8 9 10
Anxieties	**X** 1 2 3 4 5 6 7 8 9 10	**X** 1 2 3 4 5 6 7 8 9 10
Morning stiffness	0 1 2 3 4 5 6 7 **X** 9 10	**X** 1 2 3 4 5 6 7 8 9 10
Oedema	0 1 2 3 4 5 **X** 7 8 9 10	**X** 1 2 3 4 5 6 7 8 9 10
Sleeping disorder	0 1 2 3 4 5 6 7 **X** 9 10	0 1 **X** 3 4 5 6 7 8 9 10
Insecure gait impaired coordination	0 1 2 3 4 **X** 6 7 8 9 10	**X** 1 2 3 4 5 6 7 8 9 10
Pressure in the upper abdomen	0 1 2 3 4 5 6 **X** 8 9 10	**X** 1 2 3 4 5 6 7 8 9 10
Headaches	0 1 2 3 4 5 6 7 8 **X** 10	**X** 1 2 3 4 5 6 7 8 9 10
Joint aches	0 1 2 3 4 5 6 7 **X** 9 10	**X** 1 2 3 4 5 6 7 8 9 10
Swelling of lymph nodes	0 1 2 **X** 4 5 6 7 8 9 10	**X** 1 2 3 4 5 6 7 8 9 10

With this case I would also like to document that this therapy naturally also works for "outpatients", who are possibly somewhat more sceptic with regards to the therapeutic approach than "my" patients are. According to my experience, this is to be expected. The "belief" is simply irrelevant with regards to the success of a toxoplasmosis therapy. The treatment is effective and from my point of view it is also highly improbable that the state of health in patients who have been ill for such a long time as Ms X. could be improved by a placebo effect. In November 2019 she is healthy since 23 months, there has been no relapse.

14. Advances in diagnostic methods

As I have pointed out repeatedly, Toxoplasma is a real master of disguise and it is very difficult to develop a test that can safely show the existence and activity of bradyzoites. There are some scientists who are convinced of the necessity for new detection methods and who are working arduously on them. Their success is of utmost importance. If Toxoplasma-related diseases were unequivocally detectable in the laboratory, diagnostics would be significantly improved and the acceptance of toxoplasmosis therapy by doctors would surely increase as well.

I consider a new approach of the scientific group led by Professor Yolken in Baltimore to be promising. A paper on this approach has been published in June, 2018 (93). The scientists used a known detection method (a Western blot test) for the detection of Toxoplasma *proteins*, which also give proof of the presence of Toxoplasma. Of 25 patients, who were suffering from severe psychic disorders, 3 patients (8.2%) were diagnosed as positive with Toxoplasma IgG. Four times as many, 12 patients (35.3%) were then diagnosed with Toxoplasma by detection of Toxoplasma protein in their blood. The detection of these proteins seems to offer a significantly more sensitive method to diagnose toxoplasmosis than the usual available antibody tests. Until this can be used as a routine procedure, the tests will have to be examined in further studies.

The same group of scientists is currently developing another highly-sensitive method, which can detect Toxoplasma cysts in every stage of the disease. This concerns the MAG1 antigen, which occurs in great numbers inside the bradyzoite cysts and in their outer membrane.

Antibodies which are directed against this MAG1 antigen can be detected in the laboratory. The scientist could prove in mice that the amount of MAG1 antibodies detectable in the blood showed a significant correlation to the amount of bradyzoite cysts inside the brain. It was also shown that in case of negative MAG1 antibody detection, no bradyzoite cysts were found. This marker could possibly be used as a scale for a chronic infection and for the burden with bradyzoite cysts in the future. This would be a huge step for laboratory diagnostics and for affected patients even more so.

Another approach is that clues for a disturbed metabolism in patients with *Chronic Fatigue Syndrome* (CFS) are being investigated intensively. In 2016 it was proven that CFS patients share anomalies in 20 metabolic pathways of their mitochondria (60). One might picture mitochondria best as our cells' power plants. The intensity of the illness in CFS patients negatively impacts the activity of the metabolic pathways and the quantity of metabolites, which result from the mitochondria's work. This "shutdown" of the metabolism has been interpreted as a shifting of the mitochondrial metabolism into "survival mode".

Toxoplasma can also very severely affect the mitochondria (79), and the intensity of affliction is probably related to the strain of Toxoplasma which has infected the patient (65). It would be of utmost interest if the deviations in mitochondria metabolism during a chronic active toxoplasmosis might resemble those detected in ME/CFS patients, as there is strong overlap in the symptoms of both diseases. They might even be identical in some cases.

The Lymphocyte-Tranformation-Test **(LTT)** has made my work on Toxoplasmosis easier in the last months, but is not (yet) used for the diagnose of toxoplasmosis on a wider scale. It is performed by the IMD Lab in Berlin, but of course there are other labs, which can perform a Toxoplasma LTT as well. By means of this test, we can detect activity of our immune system's T-lymphocytes, which react specifically towards certain pathogens. While the immune system is dealing with certain pathogens, T-lymphocytes become specifically reactive to this pathogen, and the intensity of this reactivity can be measured pathogen-specifically.

This is measurable for about 4 weeks, and thus the LTT mirrors the current activity of pathogens. A more than threefold elevated stimulating index (SI) indicates, that specific T-cells are present in the blood and thus an active confrontation of the immune system and the tested germ takes place. A validation concerning chronic active toxoplasmosis has not yet been performed, but according to both Dr. Hopf-Seidel and my own experiences with patients suffering from a chronic active toxoplasmosis, it is most likely more sensitive than the Toxoplasma IgM.

14.1 The Toxoplasma LTT in daily use

I need to make clear that this chapter reflects only my personal experience. There are several reasons why my daily work and experience cannot be regarded as the results of a scientific study. The simplest reason is that I don't have the choice of whether or not I will prescribe treatment for a patient when I have come to the conclusion that he suffers from an active toxoplasmosis. It is my obligation to treat every patient to the best of my ability.

Since 2/2019 I have introduced the Toxoplasma LTT in my daily work. It is ordered if the symptoms listed on the checklist indicate a high risk for a chronic active toxoplasmosis and other possible reasons for the disease have been ruled out.   Unfortunately I cannot publish exact numbers here, because that could put my work close to a "study", and there might be officials who would not approve of that. So, although I am convinced that these numbers are significant, presenting them here might misrepresent my clinical experience. Nevertheless, on request I will be happy to communicate more detailed information directly to colleagues In this book, I can only give some key information:

*If a thorough exclusion of other diseases has been performed, and the Checklist Toxoplasmosis indicates a high risk for a chronic active toxoplasmosis and the Toxoplasma LTT shows a **positive** result, my experience is there is a strong chance (well above 80%) that a toxoplasmosis treatment will be a successs.*

*If a thorough exclusion of other diseases has been performed, and the Checklist Toxoplasmosis indicates a high risk for a chronic active toxoplasmosis and the Toxoplasma LTT shows a **negative** result, my experience is there is still a chance (approximately 50%) that a toxoplasmosis treatment will be successful.*

Antibody assays were of little help. Toxoplasma IgG was only elevated in some cases with positive Toxoplasma LTT, but there was no apparent correlation to the intensity of symptoms. The IgM showed negative results in every case.

In my surgery to date, the Toxoplasma IgM showed a slightly elevated result only in two (older) cases of the more than 150 patients who have undergone a successful treatment. This suggests that in chronic active toxoplasmosis the LTT is far better able to identify patients in need of a treatment than the tachyzoite - IgM antibody assay. However, LTT negative results do not allow a secure exclusion of chronic active toxoplasmosis.

In the future probably several different methods will be combined to precisely detect Toxoplasma activity. Treating doctors could screen their patients with targeted questions, and could arrange for specific laboratory diagnostics in case an active toxoplasmosis is suspected. The significance of these new diagnostic methods with regards to chronic active toxoplasmosis has not yet been decided in a formal setting.

My personal experience, although more detailed than I can present here, is only a very provisional replacement for a formal validation of Lab results in a study setting, but since institutions conducting basic research are still not very interested in the matter, this first experience is all we have to go for now. It might be a long wait until the urgently required studies are performed.

14.2. Two case documentations with positive LTT

Ms. Sabine S. age 50 years, was suffering from depression and tiredness of unknown origin for some years. In 4/2016, a close friend of her's passed away, which affected her seriously, and her health detoriated more and more. Tiredness increased, and profuse sweating set in, as well as muscular pains, exertional dispnoea, listlessness, and a concentration disorder developed. The whole disease had worsened gradually during the last three years.

In May 2019 we had a consultation and the checklist revealed a high risk for a chronic active toxoplasmosis. **Lab results: Toxoplasma IgG 64,8 IU/ml, IgM 6,06 AU/ml, Toxoplasma LTT 23,0 SI (positiv above 3).**

Due to the typical combination of symptoms and significant positive Toxoplasma LTT a combination therapy, consisting of clindamycine 3 x 300 mg, daraprim 2 x 25 mg and Calciumfolate 6,35 mg 1 x 1, was prescribed. This resulted in a good amelioration of symptoms, but the efficacy of this treatment decreased after 10 days, and the symptoms increased again. We switched to a revolving therapy:

- Pyrimethamine 25 mg 2 x 1 and Calciumfolinate 6,35 mg 1 x 1 were
  taken continuously. An antiobiotic was added, at first

- Cotrimoxazole 960 mg 2 x 1,   after 5 days this was changed to

- Clarithromycine 500 mg 2 x 1,   after 5 days this was changed to

- Clindamycine 300 mg 3 x 1,   after 5 days this was switched back to

  Cotrimoxazole 960 mg 2 x 1 again, and the whole system was repeated.

This revolving therapy resulted in a continuous improvement of all symptoms. For comment see page 216

Checklist Toxoplasmosis

Mr/Mrs. Sabine S.

Age: 50 years	**Duration**......3½......years	**Intervalls** yes / **no**
Toxoplasma	**IgG** ....64,8 IU/ml	**IgM**.................6,1 AU/ml
LTT 23,0 SI	**Date:**.................21.5.2019	**Date:** 16.7.2019
Treatment:	clindamycin 3 x 300 mg	Revolving therapy

Symptom	clindamycin 3 x 300 mg	Revolving therapy
Fatigue	0 1 2 3 4 5 6 7 **X** 9 10	0 1 **X** 3 4 5 6 7 8 9 10
Muscular pains	0 1 2 3 4 **X** 6 7 8 9 10	0 **X** 2 3 4 5 6 7 8 9 10
Concentration disorders	0 1 2 3 4 5 6 **X** 8 9 10	0 1 **X** 3 4 5 6 7 8 9 10
Sweating	0 1 2 3 4 5 6 7 8 **X** 10	0 1 **X** 3 4 5 6 7 8 9 10
Dispnoea	0 1 2 3 4 5 **X** 7 8 9 10	0 1 **X** 3 4 5 6 7 8 9 10
Listlessness	0 1 2 3 4 5 6 7 8 9 **X**	0 1 2 3 **X** 5 6 7 8 9 10
Irritability	0 1 **X** 3 4 5 6 7 8 9 10	0 **X** 2 3 4 5 6 7 8 9 10
Visual disturbance	0 1 2 3 **X** 5 6 7 8 9 10	0 1 **X** 3 4 5 6 7 8 9 10
Dizziness	0 **X** 2 3 4 5 6 7 8 9 10	**X** 1 2 3 4 5 6 7 8 9 10
Depressive moods	0 1 2 3 4 5 6 7 8 **X** 10	0 1 2 **X** 4 5 6 7 8 9 10
Anxieties	0 1 2 3 **X** 5 6 7 8 9 10	0 1 **X** 3 4 5 6 7 8 9 10
Morning stiffness	0 1 2 3 **X** 5 6 7 8 9 10	0 **X** 2 3 4 5 6 7 8 9 10
Oedema	0 1 2 3 **X** 5 6 7 8 9 10	0 **X** 2 3 4 5 6 7 8 9 10
Sleeping disorder	0 1 2 3 4 5 6 7 8 9 **X**	0 1 2 **X** 4 5 6 7 8 9 10
Insecure gait / impaired coordination	0 1 2 **X** 4 5 6 7 8 9 10	0 **X** 2 3 4 5 6 7 8 9 10
Pressure in the upper abdomen	0 1 2 3 **X** 5 6 7 8 9 10	0 1 **X** 3 4 5 6 7 8 9 10
Headaches	0 1 2 **X** 4 5 6 7 8 9 10	**X** 1 2 3 4 5 6 7 8 9 10
Joint aches	0 1 2 3 **X** 5 6 7 8 9 10	0 **X** 2 3 4 5 6 7 8 9 10
Swelling of lymph nodes	**X** 1 2 3 4 5 6 7 8 9 10	**X** 1 2 3 4 5 6 7 8 9 10

Comment: Ms. S. had been ill from a chronic active Toxoplasmosis for only 3 years, and as in other cases with a short duration of disease, most symptoms in the lower part of the checklist are not very pronounced. The Toxoplasma IgG is significant positive at 64,8 IU/ml and indicates that a tachyzoite activity has taken part recently. The Toxoplasma IgM is, at 6,06 AU/ml, not significantly increased.

In a traditional practice these results would mean, that a toxoplasmosis treatment would not be prescribed. On a closer look, negative   IgM merely show, that there is presently no significant activity of tachzoites. They don't tell us anything about bradyzoite activity, which can cause significant symptoms on its own (42).

> *The positive Toxoplasma LTT of 23,0 SI indicates, that there is a toxo-plasma activity, but as the tachyzoite-specific IgM is not significantly increseased, this activity is most likely caused by bradyzoites.*

> *Together with the result of the checklist, the significantly positive Toxoplasma LTT overruled the result of the antibody assays and justified prescribing a combination   therapy from the beginning on. This resulted in a good amelioration of symptoms. When the effect of this therapy decreased after 10 days, the significant toxoplasma LTT result backed the decision for a revolving therapy, which finally led to a very good remission of all symptoms.*

Ms. Lara P.

age 43, was suffering since her youth from various physical and psychic complaints, during several treatments in hospitals this had repeatedly been diagnosed as psychosomatic disorder. Especially pressure and pain in the upper middle abdomen, which increased after taking a meal, were very incriminating, while the gastroskopy indicated only a slight gastritis. Ultrasound and Lab results of the the pankreas were inconspicious. An acid reducing drug (Pantoprazol) was of little help. Altogether a conclusive diagnose couldn't be found and thus a satisfactory treatment could not be prescribed.

Apart from this, since at least 9 year there had been multiple musculoskeletal complaints, such as pains of the vertebral column, the knees, the finger- and toe joints, the muscles on both sides of the vertebral column and of the abdominal wall. The abdomen also showed palpable indurated (hardened) spots in the subcutaneus connective tissue. A general pain in all muscles and connective tissue could be observed.   A CT controlled therapy was only of little use, and a rheumatic disease could not be confirmed in a specialized clinic. The overall exercise capacity was significantly reduced.

At this time, there had been named already at least 20 diagnoses, for example: chronic pain syndrome with somatical and psychic symptoms, chronic generalized pain syndrome stage III, Fibromyalgic syndrome, Post traumatic stress disorder, Unstable personality disorder, Irritable stomach, Irritable bowl, reduced cardiopulmonal performance, positional vertigo.

The combination of symptoms was typical for a chronic active toxoplasmosis, however Toxoplasma IgG and IgM delivered normal results. In August, 2015 clindamycin 300 3 x 1 was prescribed for the first time. The result was a significant relief of the muscular pain and tissue pain within just one week, but the patient refused to take a combination therapy, because she was afraid of side effects. I don't blame her. It is quite understandable that a patient is sceptical regarding a diagnose which relies the presence of certain symptoms, an exclusion of other diseases and the effect of medication.

In late 2016 a pneumonia lead to a significant aggravation of all symptoms. The illness now developed in bouts with increasing symptoms every 3 or 4 weeks. In January of 2017 the toxoplasmosis checklist again showed the typical symptoms of a chronic active toxoplasmosis, but since the lab results still showing inconspicious results, the patient was still sceptical about a toxoplasmosis treatment.

In Juli, 2019 the Toxoplasma LTT was performed for the first time, showing 4,9 SI (positive above 3), while the antibody assays were still negative. Due to the positive result of the LTT and a significant result of the checklist a decision for a toxoplasmosis treatment was made.

Therapy: I prescribed Daraprim 2 x 25 mg, Calciumfolate 6,35 mg 1 x 1 and Co-trimoxazole 960 mg 2 x 1. This had a very positive effect, but after approximately 14 days, the symptoms increased again. At this point, I switched to a revolving therapy (see also pp. 188 / 189), which resulted in a continuous, significant improvement. The therapy was prescribed as follows:

- Pyrimethamine 25 mg (Daraprim) 2 x 1 and Calciumfolinate 6,35 mg
  1 x 1 were taken continuously.   An antiobiotic was added, at first

- Co-trimoxazol 960 mg mg 2 x 1, after 5 days this was changed to

- Clindamycine 300 mg 3 x 1, after 5 days this was to

- Clarithromycine 500 mg 2 x 1, after 5 days this was changed to co-
  trimoxazol again, and the whole system was repeated again.

This medication resulted in a continuous, significant improvement
without any renewed loss of efficacy. After 6 weeks of continuous
therapy the patient was almost free of symptoms, and we switched to a
relapse prophylaxes with 3 treatment days a week for one month and
with 2 treatment days for another month. In the second month we
switched only between Co-trimoxazole and Clarithromycine from one
week to another, as clindamycin began to cause side effects.

Comment: The documentation gives only a small insight, how the
strongly expressed symptoms literally overshadowed the whole life of
the patient, and how difficult the search for this diagnose had been.
Until we came to this point, the patient unfortunately had to endure
several major setbacks – but their psychic problems were by no means
the origin of this disease.

The benefit of the Toxoplasma LTT is plain to see, for without its
positive result I doubtlessly would not have been able to convince the
patient that a toxoplasma treatment would be necessary. The benefit
of the revolving therapy is such that, without this treament, a
successful therapy would most likely not have been possible.

Checklist Toxoplasmosis

Mr/Mrs. Lara P.

Age:....42...years **Duration**......9........years   **Intervalls**   **yes** / no

Toxoplasma   **IgG** ....0 IU/ml   **IgM**...................0 AU/ml

LTT 4,9 SI   **Date:**.................14.5.2019   **Date:** 27.8.2019

Treatment: clindamycin 3 x 300 mg   Revolving therapy

Symptom	clindamycin 3 x 300 mg	Revolving therapy
Fatigue	0 1 2 3 4 5 6 7 8 9 **X**	**X** 1 2 3 4 5 6 7 8 9 10
Muscular pains	0 1 2 3 4 5 6 7 **X** 9 10	**X** 1 2 3 4 5 6 7 8 9 10
Concentration disorders	0 1 2 3 4 5 6 7 8 **X** 10	0 1 **X** 3 4 5 6 7 8 9 10
Sweating	0 1 2 3 4 **X** 6 7 8 9 10	0 1 **X** 3 4 5 6 7 8 9 10
Dispnoea	0 1 2 3 4 5 6 **X** 8 9 10	0 **X** 2 3 4 5 6 7 8 9 10
Listlessness	0 1 2 3 4 5 6 7 8 9 **X**	0 **X** 2 3 4 5 6 7 8 9 10
Irritability	0 1 2 3 4 5 6 7 8 9 **X**	0 1 **X** 3 4 5 6 7 8 9 10
Visual disturbance*	1 2 3 4 5 **X** 7 8 9 10	**X** 1 2 3 4 5 6 7 8 9 10
Dizziness	0 1 2 3 4 5 6 **X** 8 9 10	**X** 1 2 3 4 5 6 7 8 9 10
Depressive moods	0 1 **X** 3 4 5 6 7 8 9 10	0 **X** 2 3 4 5 6 7 8 9 10
Anxieties**	0 1 2 3 4 5 6 7 8 9 **X**	0 1 2 3 4 5 **X** 7 8 9 10
Morning stiffness	0 1 2 3 4 5 6 7 **X** 9 10	0 **X** 2 3 4 5 6 7 8 9 10
Oedema	0 1 2 3 **X** 5 6 7 8 9 10	0 1 **X** 3 4 5 6 7 8 9 10
Sleeping disorder ***	1 2 3 4 5 6 7 8 9 **X**	0 1 2 3 **X** 5 6 7 8 9 10
Insecure gait / impaired coordination	0 1 2 3 **X** 5 6 7 8 9 10	**X** 1 2 3 4 5 6 7 8 9 10
Pressure in the upper abdomen	0 1 2 3 4 5 **X** 7 8 9 10	0 **X** 2 3 4 5 6 7 8 9 10
Headaches	0 1 2 3 4 5 6 7 **X** 9 10	0 **X** 2 3 4 5 6 7 8 9 10
Joint aches	0 1 2 3 4 5 6 7 **X** 9 10	0 **X** 2 3 4 5 6 7 8 9 10
Swelling of lymph nodes	0 1 2 3 4 5 6 7 **X** 9 10	0 **X** 2 3 4 5 6 7 8 9 10

* Ms P. also had burning sensations of the eyes   ** Ms P suffers from an anxiety disorder   *** Nykturia improved significantly, from 8-10 times to 2-3 times.

15. The reactions of the scientific world

Reactions have been rather sparing at first. You might have already noticed that I represent a minority view in the medical world, and, believe me, that has never been my intention. Still, I soon realized that I urgently needed "allies" and thus went to search for them as soon as my work had been finished. In January 2017, after 1½ years of intensive work this was finally the case. I was optimistic that I would at least be able to convince some of my colleagues and could possibly initiate a research project at a German university, something which I had been working towards the whole time. This optimism soon gave way to a significant disillusionment, since the response was just barely above "zero".   Apart from my practice associate and *one* further internist, almost nobody was interested in the topic.

I initially sent about 20 copies of my finding to universities by post, but only received an answer from my home university in Bochum and later from the university of Münster. The other universities didn't even send an acknowledgment of receipt.

I also sent mail all over Germany to further universities, medical societies and medical institutions where their main fields of work and research gave me reason to hope, that they could be interested in my work. The response remained low, but I received positive answers from Prof. Scheibenbogen of the Charité Berlin, who does intensive research on Chronic Fatigue Syndrome, as well as from Prof. Schäfer of Marburg University, who leads the department for rare and unrecognised diseases and this encouraged me to go on. Still, the few answers show that there is very little medical interest in toxoplasmosis in Germany. This is hard to understand, as our infection rate is at least 50% (88).

In contrast to that, the affected patients were very interested. The work could be downloaded free of charge from www.fatigatio.de, the website of an initiative that supports patients who are suffering from Chronic Fatigue (CFS). Soon websites in English will be available.

Thankfully, the work was now also found by affected patients, some of whom I could help myself, and others treated by their own practitioners. This was a very pleasant success, but compared to the probably very high number affected, only a drop in the ocean, and a broader acceptance among medical colleagues seemed to be in the far future.

In autumn 2017, the English translation of my work was completed. Now I could get in contact with scientists who had done decisive groundwork in this field and on whose findings my work is based. This yielded the first real success. In an open and friendly e-mail conversation, Professor Jaroslav Flegr from Prague answered in great detail and made further scientific material (30) available to me. This kept me going for the time being, but it was by no means the clinical study I was hoping for.

During my research in spring 2017, I came across very interesting work by Prof. Vernon Carruthers (21), who leads a laboratory at the University of Michigan working on a new drug that can disturb the metabolism of bradyzoites at a decisive point. It is possible that an effective drug can be developed within the next years that might be effective against bradyzoite cysts. In the treatment of toxoplasmosis this would be a big step forward.

You can also read about his research in 16.6 on p. 232. I sent him a detailed email and my work as a PDF, and received a very friendly and detailed answer a few weeks later. He had read my work, was very interested and confirmed that my scientific reasoning had been correct. He also evaluated the interpretation of my results in a positive way. Prof. Carruthers offered to put me in contact with his colleague Prof. Yolken from John Hopkins Hospital, and I gladly agreed.

John Hopkins Medical School in Baltimore incorporates a university and hospitals, and is world-renowned for state-of-the-art medicine and research. It is one of the best hospitals in the USA. It is there that Prof. Robert Yolken has been conducting intensive research for years on psychic and neurological illnesses caused by Toxoplasma gondii. He and his department can look back on 172 publications in scientific magazines, which is a very significant contribution to medical research. He had already realised years ago that our available laboratory values exhibit a wide diagnostic gap with regards to bradyzoites. To overcome this, he has developed new laboratory methods, which also enable the detection of bradyzoites inside their cysts. This was published 6 in June, 2018 in an article (93, see also pp. 209/ 210).

Prof. Yolken is well-known to me, since I have quoted many of his scientific findings in my work and in this book (22, 81, 82, 92, 93, 94). I just had not contacted him personally. The question got a whole new dynamic now, since Prof. Yolken reacted positively towards my findings. He asked whether I still had blood samples from my patients?! I unfortunately did not have any, because my case collection is not a study in the conventional sense and frozen samples are not available.

A possible collaboration with such a renowned research department exceeded my expectations, and I was willing to take any effort to make this chance a success. The study would require blood samples from patients in whom I had detected and treated chronic active toxoplasmosis. The blood samples had to be taken before and after therapy. I would then send these to Baltimore together with the previous laboratory results and the corresponding questionnaires.

A short phone call with the laboratory doctor Dr. med. Molitor from the Hygiene Institute Gelsenkirchen [an institute for laboratory medicine] showed that the hygiene institute would be pleased to centrifuge the blood samples for us, so that the blood plasma could be frozen. *I would like to express my gratitude to you for this friendly support among colleagues.*

If in Baltimore, by using the new laboratory methods bradyzoite activity could be demonstrated in my patients' serum, and this activity then shown to be reduced by therapy, it would support my diagnostic approach, and it would also demonstrate that the laboratory values developed by Prof Yolken were appropriate to diagnose a patient's chronically active toxoplasmosis, and probably also that they are more sensitive than previously available values. Perhaps in the medium term, this could finally be the impetus for major clinical studies, which could then deliver definitive evidence.

It would be a study this time, and a license from the Ethics Committee of the Medical Association Münster would be required before beginning. I was cautiously optimistic of getting permission, because my diagnoses or the therapies I had prescribed would not be dependent on participation in this study and could obviously not be influenced by subsequent laboratory tests. All data related to the treatments would also be sent anonymously to the USA. Disadvantages for my patients would certainly be excluded.

It turned out that it is most difficult to get such permission. I was still in negotiation with the Ethics Committee when something very odd and uncommon happened. The freezer in the basement which contained the samples of about 20 patients broke down in May 2019 and this destroyed the samples.

I was really downcast, because these samples were potentially of high scientific worth, and it had cost not a little energy to do this additional work and to negotiate with the Ethical Commission. Confronted with these obstacles I decided to cancel this project, and I am very sorry for that. Please keep in mind that I have to run a practise. This leaves little room for other projects, and continuing would surely have over-stretched my powers. Unfortunately, by the time of this writing in October, 2019 I haven't found a medical department interested in performing a clinical study about the bradyzoites' role in chronic active toxoplasmosis or which would just support my work. They are just not interested.

In general practice, bradyzoite activity is still, in contradiction to basic research, not regarded as a problem, and thus it is still assumed that our antibody assays reflecting only the tachyzoites' activity would be sufficient to diagnose an active toxoplasmosis securely.

That these tests were designed at a time when the antigen shift during the conversion from tachyzoites to bradyzoites was still unknown, does not, for some reason, disturb this view.

By October 2019 I found contact with other interested doctors through patients who are spread all over Germany and who have downloaded my work and/or have read my book. Some have already familiarised themselves with this field and my treated patients. Things are moving slowly, but then medicine has never been known for rapid progress.

The latest development is that I was invited to a congress of the German Borreliosis Society in October 2019. The presentation of my work was accepted with interest, and I am confident that some of these colleagues will consider a chronic active toxoplasmosis more often in their daily work. I met an open-minded audience and assume that the reason for this is that doctors who deal with borreliosis have to face diagnostic difficulties regularly. They are also well aware that presumably "latent" infections can be a much more serious risk to our health than is widely assumed, and chronic active toxoplasmosis is surely a striking example of that.

16. FAQ = frequently asked questions

16.1. Can symptom intensities change?

Yes, and that is quite often the case. In about one out of five of my patients (cases 8, 11, 13, 16 and 23) the symptoms showed an interval-like progression. This means that the affected patients had phases with fewer symptoms, lasting between 1 and 4 weeks, alternating with severe disease phases lasting up to about 10 days. Chronic active toxoplasmosis is more difficult to diagnose in this form, but the symptoms tend to be alleviated rapidly and particularly well by the therapies. Therefore, I suppose that in such progressions the immune system of those affected is close to regaining control over the disease in the symptom-poor phases, but only just close to doing so.

Therapy should also be considered in the case of an interval-like course. The quality of life is already clearly impaired and there is a risk, that the disease will switch to severe continuous symptoms, if the performance of the immune system diminishes due to exhaustion or stressful factors such as surgery, pneumonia, serious viral infections or severe mental stress. Once an active toxoplasmosis has switched to a continuous disease, the immune system often seems unable to regain control, and symptoms tend to increase significantly.

Beware: Fever episodes or chills are not explicitly the typical symptoms in a chronically active toxoplasmosis, even in the case of an interval-shaped progression. This symptom may indicate a spreading of pathogens in the blood stream (septicaemia) and require a thorough differential diagnosis.

16.2. Are there other lab values that indicate chronic active toxoplasmosis?

I found only very few deviations in laboratory results, whether these tests were initiated by me or by a specialist clinic. Only the muscle enzyme creatine kinase (CK) indicated in some cases a slightly increased value on an impairment of the muscles, but this is nonspecific and does not allow precise conclusions about the cause. Likewise, a slight increase in erythrocyte sedimentation that I have observed in some cases was unspecific in origin. Further deviations did not show up. New laboratory techniques (see chapters 14, p. 209) are promising, but not all of them are available in Europe, and they have still to undergo a validation.

In my daily work, I have introduced the Toxoplasma LTT (performed by the IMD lab, Berlin), and my personal experience is so far very positive. In my experience, it is far more sensitive in detecting a chronic active toxoplasmosis than the Toxoplasma IgM. The exact sensitivity and specificity in diagnosing a chronic active toxoplasmosis is still to be validated in a study. In my work, I found some patients who tested negative with Toxoplasma LTT, but suffered from a chronic active toxoplasmosis, and who could be treated with success. Nevertheless, the majority of patients who tested positive with the toxoplasma LTT reacted very well to a toxoplasmosis treatment (see pp. 212 / 213).

For many reasons I have come to believe that chronically active toxoplasmosis cannot be reliably diagnosed or excluded with currently available laboratory data.

16.3.   Should I have my Toxoplasma antibodies determined?

This should only be considered if there are clear symptoms of active toxoplasmosis and if other diseases have been excluded.   Remember, *only tachyzoite-specific antibodies can currently be determined.* A positive IgG detection in these cases proves that you are a carrier of toxoplasmosis, and that the symptoms *could* be triggered by this.

A positive IgM would prove active toxoplasmosis in need of treatment, with the serious limitation that Toxoplasma IgM has been shown to be very unreliable. In the case of a negative test result it may be that an infection with Toxoplasma gondii took place a long time ago, the antibodies have decreased sharply and the test result has become negative, although Toxoplasma in the form of bradyzoites may still be present and active.

According to my observations, no tachyzoite antibodies are detectable in about 40% of patients who are suffering from chronic active toxoplasmosis. Therefore, it cannot automatically be concluded from a negative antibody test that the symptoms of a patient are not caused by Toxoplasma and that treatment is not required. (see Chapter 11.3, p.161)

So concluding, the antibody-based assays are unfortunately spreading uncertainty because of their unreliability. If you have no symptoms of active toxoplasmosis, determining Toxoplasma antibodies is certainly not useful, except in the case of pregnancy - see 16.8. from p. 234.

16.4. Am I immune to Toxoplasma after an initial infection?

It has been known since 1967 that cells from lymph nodes and spleens of hamsters infected with toxoplasmosis were able to protect other hamsters from toxoplasma infection (32). It was concluded that cell-mediated immunity developed in an initial Toxoplasma infection. Antibodies had almost no protective effect.

I am not aware of systematic studies on humans with regards to such an immunity to Toxoplasma.

It is also a problem that atypical mixed forms of the known Toxoplasma strains, which are significantly more aggressive than the previously known Toxoplasma strains have been detected in Germany (43, 72), and this might happen worldwide. Whether a previous infection with a "normal" Toxoplasma strain has a protective effect on infection with these mixed forms is currently still completely unclear. The assumption that an endured toxoplasmosis leaves a safe immunity against further Toxoplasma infections is not proven. Possibly a protective effect provided by immunity takes place only when the human is infected with the same Toxoplasma strain again.

In any case, I cannot recommend consumption of unprocessed meat products or close contact to an ill cat, trusting to a possible immunity.

16.5. Is my cat a threat to my health?

Regrettably, yes. If the cat is not kept inside and fed only with cooked meat, it will sooner or later be infected with toxoplasma, and thus cat owners do have an increased risk of becoming infected (88), but:

- It is possible that you have already been infected with toxoplasma, whether or not you are a cat owner. An older cat often distributes fewer oocysts in case of renewed infections (33) and thus the risk of infecting humans is reduced a little with time. Unfortunately, as has been mentioned, we are at the time not able to diagnose a Toxoplasma infection securely or explicitly to rule it out.

- A transmission of Toxoplasma through a direct contact with a recently infected cat via Oocysts is only *one* way of becoming infected. Bradyzoite cysts in uncooked meat is a more frequent source of infection (14), and oocysts can also be transferred on vegetables or in water (4).

- It can be concluded that cats are the key factor in spreading this disease and the risk to cat owners is increased. It may well be that a cat owner, who has become a toxoplasma carrier, might not have been infected by her own cat, but by another one, which had spread oocysts in the environment. You might have a second look on chapters 6.1 – 6.3.

> *Since you might have already been infected, there is no point in abandoning a cat, but you might think one more time about getting one, especially a young one, and especially if children will come in close contact with it. Keeping the cat inside and feeding it only cooked meat reduces the risk.*

16.6. Is there a therapy that kills Toxoplasma completely?

Unfortunately, such a therapy is not yet available, but research is being performed on drugs that can disrupt the metabolism of bradyzoites and probably kill them. Currently, a research group led by Professor Carruthers at the University of Michigan has investigated a drug that inhibits a key enzyme in bradyzoite metabolism and thus eradicate them (21).

However, the active ingredient cannot be used therapeutically because it cannot penetrate the "blood-brain-barrier" and is therefore ineffective in the central nervous system. If this problem can be solved and clinical studies carried out, then in the future an active substance could be available which might kill bradyzoites effectively, and this would bring us very close to a complete cure for toxoplasmosis.

There are also broader efforts that are being exerted by several different research teams, as reflected in a recent review (57), to find drugs that are effective against Toxoplasma tissue cysts and thus against bradyzoits, but most of them are in the early stages of testing. So the tissue cysts are, until today, a "save haven" (76) for Toxoplasma – and we will need some more time until we can them attack more effectively. Only then we will be able to heal this disease completely and to prevent a renewed Toxoplasma activity securely.

16.7. Is my immune system burdened by toxoplasmosis therapy?

Many people are aware that overuse of antibiotics over years can lead to more and more persistent infections. This is often interpreted as a weakening of the immune system, but rather it is due to developed resistance and damage to our microbiome by antibiotics. Please re-read "The risks of antibiotics" starting on p.86.

The immune system of patients with chronic active toxoplasmosis is severely affected by the parasite's activity and many of these patients suffer from frequent infections. These occur significantly less often after a successful toxoplasmosis therapy, so the immune system rather benefits here.

Only in very few cases have I seen a decrease in white blood cells as a side-effect of toxoplasmosis therapy as shown by appropriate blood count monitoring. That's one of the reasons why I keep insisting on laboratory controls and close monitoring by the general practitioner.

In every cases where lab tests showed a problem, therapies were interrupted immediately. In all cases the blood count normalized within a few days after discontinuing the medication, and in no case was there a permanent impairment of the immune system. Unfortunately, a safe avoidance of any side-effects is only possible if you completely refrain from a toxoplasmosis therapy.

16.8. Toxoplasma antibody determination in pregnancy

I would like to recommend that women who are planning on becoming pregnant seek advice from their gynaecologist. A detailed article on toxoplasmosis in pregnancy was published in 2001 in Deutsches Ärzteblatt and the article is available at www.ärzteblatt.de. An internet search will reveal other articles in English or other languages.

Tests are used during pregnancy to detect a primary infection at an early stage. They are well suited for this, since in an initial infection Tachyzoites are likely to appear in the blood in such a high number that tachyzoite-specific antibodies become detectable.

It is certain that toxoplasma damage to the embryo is unlikely if Toxoplasma antibodies are detectable in the mother's blood before pregnancy. The immune system has by then developed an increased preparedness, so that a renewed Toxoplasma infection during pregnancy does not pose a great risk for embryonic damage. Of course, you should avoid another Toxoplasma infection during pregnancy because there are at least 3 Toxoplasma strains and the protective effect after an initial infection may relate only to the Toxoplasma strain that caused the initial infection. Information on avoiding Toxoplasma infections can be found in chapter 6.2. from p.45.

If no Toxoplasma antibodies are present in the mother's blood before pregnancy, but then become detectable during pregnancy, this indicates an initial infection which, if left untreated, can endanger the child at all stages of pregnancy.

The risk is aggravated by the fact that an initial infection during pregnancy causes little or no warning symptoms in about 75% of cases. That is why gynaecologists and paediatricians often recommend several tests during pregnancy for women without symptoms.

My frequent criticism of the reliability of Toxoplasma gondii laboratory tests relates primarily to the chronic active form of toxoplasmosis, in which the bradyzoites play a major role and whose activity cannot be detected by our tachyzoite-specific laboratory data.

If antibodies are not detectable prior to pregnancy, regular screening for Toxoplasma antibodies during pregnancy is a useful measure as the woman has probably never suffered from an initial infection. In these cases, an increase in antibodies proves an initial infection, and it is absolutely indisputable that treatment should be started as soon as possible to prevent infection of the child.

Consequently, a free of charge Toxoplasma screening for pregnant women is offered in Austria and other countries since 1975. Early treatment of primary infections during pregnancy in the last 20 years has reduced the incidence of new born toxoplasma infections in Austria from about 78 per 10,000 births to less than 1 per 10,000 births (67).

16.9. Does the therapy work for all?

Unfortunately, no. There are about 10% of patients who have symptoms of active toxoplasmosis who do not benefit from Toxoplasma treatment and another 10-20% whose symptoms improve only partially. That's about 20-30% of all patients. This is an estimate based on my personal experience and only a clinical trial could provide more accurate results.

Often, these patients have been ill for a very long time, and it is conceivable that the cyst burden in these patients is so high that our current therapies cannot improve the situation. According to recent research, it is also possible that in such cases the mitochondrial metabolism might be disturbed by the Toxoplasma (80). Such disorders may be more commonly triggered by type I and III Toxoplasma (65).

Combinations with other diseases or deficiencies could in some cases explain a poor or non-existent effect of the therapy and this is discussed in Chapter 7 from page 61 on. Finally, it might be possible that a disease or even a combination of diseases imitates a chronic active Toxoplasmosis in every aspect.

All patients with symptoms of toxoplasmosis must be aware that there is some uncertainty about whether the therapy will be effective until the end of the first 7-10 days of clindamycin therapy. There is a strong chance (about 70%) that Toxoplasma is the reason for their disease **when a thorough differential diagnosis has been performed and when the checklist shows a significant result.** A positive Toxoplasma LTT increases this chance and thus the chance of a successful treatment further, to well above 80% (see pp 212 / 213).

16.10. Which doctors can treat toxoplasmosis?

In principle, every doctor can familiarize himself/herself with this field and treat chronic active toxoplasmosis and general practitioners, internists and rheumatologists are particularly situated to do so.

Some doctors regard it as problematic that the therapy of an active toxoplasmosis is initially a *healing attempt (taking a course of action on the basis of deduction rather than relying on a test result)*. Even with the utmost care, it sometimes cannot be absolutely proven that a chronically active toxoplasmosis is the cause of the disease before the start of therapy. If other conditions have been excluded with a thorough history and differential diagnosis (see Chapter 7 p. 61), the checklist allows a risk assessment of active toxoplasmosis, but it does not provide definitive evidence. However, diagnostic uncertainty persists only for the first 7-10 days, because if initial treatment with clindamycin is successful, the subsequent combination therapy is almost always successful.

Nevertheless, not every doctor wants to prescribe such a healing attempt, and he can continue to rely solely on the laboratory diagnostics and thus simply reject a treatment attempt because of negative test results. That is regrettable, but is his professional decision. Unfortunately, other than my case collection, there is no clinical study that investigated the frequency of chronically active toxoplasmosis in negative IgM or completely unobtrusive laboratory tests. As long as this is not yet available, many doctors will insist on the lab findings so far. A positive LTT result may help to convince them to prescribe a toxoplasmosis treatment in some cases – unfortunately there are still some cases in which even the LTT shows a negative result although a chronic active toxoplasmosis takes place.

Carefully documented testimonials have always had a certain significance in medicine, but observations in a practitioner's surgery currently hardly play any role.

New insights are actually only obtained from large medical departments, with the research priorities being set by those who pay for the necessary and very expensive studies. Unfortunately, it may take years before a clinical study on chronically active toxoplasmosis is finally completed, because research funds often flow only when new drugs might be established in the market.

I am convinced that it is medically absolutely reasonable that a doctor tries to help a patient with this therapeutic approach in carefully considered cases. As far as possible, I have explained this through a thorough technical argumentation and case studies and formulated a decision aid with the checklist. Our patients need our help today, not in possibly 10 or 15 years, when new laboratory methods have been validated and widely accepted.

If the criteria are met, some doctors will give this therapy approach a chance, because ultimately all that matters is that we want to help our patients. The decision to undertake a toxoplasmosis treatment is in many cases a difficult one, so it is understandable that doctors will need some time and serious consideration to come to a conclusion.

16.11. Is the treatment of an active toxoplasmosis covered by health insurance?

The answer will be specific for countries or insurance companies, so please check with your doctor and your insurance. In an ideal world, a toxoplasma treatment as well as the regular checks for toxoplasma antibodies during pregnancy should be covered everywhere. In the long run, a declining infection rate worldwide would set free a huge financial as well as health benefit (31).

In Germany the treatment is covered by statutory health insurance, but there are catches. The treatments are time consuming and the drugs are not cheap. In Germany the medication budget for patients with statutory health insurance is quite tight, to put it very nicely. This point in particular is a major problem for many German physicians because it places them at a high risk in the form of potential recourse claims. More in chapter 17 from page 243 onwards.

16.12 Why is chronic active Toxoplasmosis different from acute Toxoplasmosis?

In acute Toxoplasmosis, the disease is caused by Toxoplasma in form of tachyzoits, which multiply fast and invade and blast host cells, whereas in the course of chronic active Toxoplasmosis, the disease is caused predominantly by a chronic increased activitiy of *Toxoplasma - bradyzoits within their cysts*, without blasting their host cells. It is more difficult to diagnose, especially because the methods in use were developed to detect activity of *Toxoplasma - tachyzoits outside the cysts and host cells*. The characteristics of the resulting clinical pictures show remarkable differencies; I would suggest to use an own abbreviation for chronic active toxoplasmosis: CATOX.

16.13 What happens if I have undiagnosed symptoms and I want my doctor to investigate toxoplasmosis?

Of course, your doctor *is* familiar with toxoplasmosis, but very few doctors are familiar with research which shows that an infection producing symptoms doesn't necessarily result in a positive test result. Even fewer know of the use of the LLT test.

If you are in the unfortunate position of having severe symptoms of exhaustion, unclear muscle pains, poor concentration, poor performance and shortness of breath, sweating, depressive moods, aggressive behavioural changes and anxiety *and your physician has tried every test and procedure without finding a conclusive diagnosis,* then you might wish to bring up the possibility of toxoplasmosis. The response from your physician might be to point out that the relevant test has been performed and has shown no infection.

The reluctance of your physician to probe further is to be respected. He or she is relying on medical information and traditions and isn't trying to be obstructive. At that point I would recommend to ask your doctor for a Toxoplasma LTT. He might not be familiar with the LTT, but it should not be a big problem to find a lab that is able to perform this test. The Lab will need about 10 to 14 days to deliver the LTT result, and that would be the right time to have another appointment with your physician, bringing your completed checklist with you.

As you are having trouble with fatigue, listlessness and concentration, you might need help in both digesting all I have written as well as in presenting this information to a busy physician. Your husband or your wife or a friend, especially if that friend is a nurse or other qualified person, can be invaluable in helping you.

Your doctor is used to a ten-minute consultation with patients under normal circumstances, and a 30-or-more-minute interview to fill out an unfamiliar checklist is difficult to justify, or to bill to an insurance body. You need to be proactive here. Talk about all of your symptoms with your friend and then determine for yourself what ratings you would give each symptom and fill out the checklist.

If the Toxoplasma LTT shows a positive result that corresponds to your symptoms on the checklist you have ready for your doctor, he or she might already agree to a therapy.

If the LTT delivers a negative result, your doctor might be in a bit of a quandary. He or she really wants to help you, but the new information that toxoplasma can be active despite negative lab results (even the LTT is not perfect) is difficult to grasp quickly. You might ask him to read this book; it is based on basic research in order to be able to convince even sceptic physicians. I have quoted the relevant sources, so that your doctor can follow the argumentation. If your doctor is too busy to read the whole book, copies of the pages 33 – 42, 49 – 60 and 211 – 220 might be sufficient to convince him or her.

Please keep in mind that you are asking your doctor to spend a large amount of precious time reading about a topic he might not find to be relevant in the beginning, so give him some days to process the new information. He might not be too happy to be confronted with such an unusual request, but hopefully he will take the chance to help you (as well as probably other patients as well).

If your doctor prescribes you a toxoplasmosis treatment, you can help him or her tremendously by filling out a checklist *every week.* It is very difficult to monitor the progression of the therapy without meticiously recording the symptoms. This information is extremely valuable to your doctor, as he is the one who is responsible for therapeutical decisions, and he urgently needs information about the development of your symptoms.

> *Above all, remember that your objective is to get well again, and working with your doctor is critical in examining your symptoms. This is new territory for both of you, and working together, you and your doctor can heal you.*

17. On my own behalf

A lot of this chapter is specific to the German health care system, and in order not to be misunderstood, I regard our system as a very important achievement for the whole of society. Nearly everybody has health insurance. The downside is that a certain tendency to *set tight budgets for everything* is creating a lot of problems for the working doctor and his patients. In Germany this is highly political and for other countries it might serve as a warning not to overdo bureaucracy.

This is also about the education of young doctors and the future of GP care in Germany, which currently is in a bad situation. Also, the limitations of the freedom of medical treatment, which may have disadvantages for patients suffering from chronic active toxoplasmosis, must be mentioned here.

As in any other profession, a doctor has to be constantly ready to learn. The information gathered by patients, the experiences they have with their illnesses, effects and side-effects of medications and much more add to the experience of the doctor, *if he or she cares to listen.*

In a patient interview (the anamnesis) physicians have to run through all the information that comes from the patient, process it through an internal medical "filter" and further clarify matters with interim questions. This is called "active listening" and it is an essential learning content for students doing internships in our practice. Good nonverbal communication is often underestimated, but it is also extremely important. At the same time, it is important to document as completely as possible and to develop initial strategies on how to proceed diagnostically and help the patient.

That sounds, and is, complicated and therefore time consuming and exhausting. However, the time and effort required for these interviews is well spent as the information gained is the crucial basis for medical work.

In my experience, patients are highly motivated to contribute to the cure, especially if they are taken seriously. Nobody goes to the doctor, "because it is so entertaining there". A doctor can gain much, often crucial information from such patient discussions. Care, attention to the patient, empathy, knowledge and experience are necessary. Our interns are fully involved in such discussions and are sensitive. I think we will get good young doctors who are technicians and human.

They internalize hundreds of disease patterns during their studies and this knowledge is extremely important for a good diagnosis. Only with a good medical history and a precise knowledge of many clinical pictures is a sensible preselection of the necessary examinations possible. The sole unwinding and examination of extensive technical measures often does not lead to diagnosis, especially if the disease leaves no clear mark in the laboratory. This is far more often the case than one would expect, not only in the case of chronic active toxoplasmosis.

During my own training, I was often impressed with the grasp of my older colleagues who attached great importance to the details of the medical history and good physical examination.

I also learned from them not to trust technical examination results unconditionally and, in case of doubt to put the patient at the centre of attention rather than just blindly giving technology credence. As a human, everybody has the "antennas" for it and can learn to use them. This is the attitude that characterizes my work as a general practitioner, and ultimately brought me on the trail of Toxoplasma gondii.

The health burden of active toxoplasmosis in terms of pain, fatigue, concentration disorders, limited resilience, mental stress and much more is unpredictable and, given the probably very high number of people affected, "immense" is not an exaggeration. The financial burden on society and the health system from this disease is likely to be very high given the frequency of illnesses, sick leave and inpatient care.

Health economists could calculate this on the basis of larger studies and the sum would be certainly frightening. The current cost of drugs for a complete treatment of chronic active toxoplasmosis, which is to be borne by health insurance in Germany is about €210 (about $US 245) for a sulfadiazine combined therapy up to €480 (about $US 535) for a Rovamycin mono-therapy. With prolonged therapy or other medications more resources may be needed.

Just to mention another, similarly serious disease, a Lyme disease treatment by antibiotics infusions, for example 30 days Ceftriaxone 2.0g daily, currently costs about €750 ($US835). It is worth the money, especially considering that these people are very seriously ill and that healing is often possible.

However, if patients with statutory health insurance are affected, in Germany such treatments cause are a high cost risk for physicians in private practice due to tight drug budgets. At present, in a general medical practice, the "benchmark" for a "statutory health insurance patient" per quarter up to the age of 15 is €20, from age 16 to age 49 it is around €36. From age 50 to age 64 it is about €89 and from the age of 65 onwards it is about €162.

This is expected to be sufficient for the drug prescriptions for 3 months and the doctor is responsible and ultimately liable. Therefore, the "benchmarks" also act like budgets and consequently physicians in private practice are constantly and intentionally under a considerable "savings pressure". In daily work, this can lead to nerve-wrecking conflicts, but it becomes a real nightmare when the average drug expenditure per patient exceeds these amounts and you as a doctor get a claim from the government for recourse.

It is also not possible to apply for previous authorization for certain therapies, which is why a doctor in Germany sometimes has to take real financial risks if he wants to treat his statutory insured patients well. This is a very significant point of annoyance of doctors with the current system.

Nevertheless, the statutory health insurance funds and the politicians are so convinced of this system that they accept heavy restrictions on the freedom of medical treatment, and thus discourage the next generation of general practitioners. I do not have the words to describe how harmful this system is to the resident physicians and ultimately to patient care.

It is also not easy for the GPs to take any time for the necessary detailed differential diagnosis, interviews and follow ups. In my experience, a total of at least 2 to 4 hours of time is required for one complete toxoplasmosis diagnosis and treatment.

Unfortunately, the medical discussion is little appreciated in many health care systems, as those responsible believe more in technical investigations. The regulations, which are in Germany are tailor-made for health insurance, and the decreasing number of general practitioners will inevitably lead to some doctors simply not being able to take the necessary time. In addition, it is unfortunately also conceivable that the tight drug budgets can adversely affect therapeutic decisions. You might imagine that it is sheer nonsense to exert a strong budgetary and recourse pressure on the general practitioners while hoping that more young doctors will complete general medical education to become GP's. That's just a shame, and it is threatening to ruin this really wonderful profession.

Here is another concrete cause for this problem in, for example, Hessen, a predominately rural German state. The largest city in Hessen is Frankfurt-am-main. There is a shortage of primary care physicians in rural areas in particular. In 2018, however, a case of repayment to state insurance was being made public again. Two Hessian country doctors were sentenced to pay a higher 5-digit reimbursement because they had made "too many" home visits. Their "crime" was they look after many older patients who can no longer come to the practice. Being less committed in their work would not have hurt these colleagues financially. *What madness.*

Such financial recourse can be assessed over several quarters for up to 2 years. Young doctors are watching this very closely and I am sure that the damage caused by such procedures cannot be remedied by a start-up loan, rent-free practice rooms or similar measures.

In about 5 years (about 2024), even primary care medicine in cities will probably be so thinned out that we will inevitably get worse care and a significant cost increase through more hospital stays, because hospital outpatient clinics or online consultations will certainly not be able to replace missing family doctors.

The positive aspect is that many doctors continue to practice their profession with commitment and joy, despite these constraints and regressive mechanisms, and I count myself one of them. I have not received any recourse claims for toxoplasmosis treatment *yet*, but I am prepared for it.

As a whole, the conditions for GP's in Germany hinder an effective treatment in some aspects. *Eventually*, this will be recognized in the next few years and the restrictions on medical treatment freedom and budgeting will be eliminated, along with demands for recourse. Another useful effect would be, that the lack of general practitioners could be counteracted effectively in this way.

18. Conclusions

It is undisputed that in Germany at least 50% of the population are infected with Toxoplasma gondii, and worldwide an infection rate of about 30% to 60% is estimated. Contrary to previous assumptions, active toxoplasmosis can also lead to serious illnesses in people with normal immune systems, and it is far more common than previously thought.

Our immune system regulates microorganisms and usually keeps them in check so that we do not get sick. However, Toxoplasma can exhaust our immune system and sometimes even control it, with severe consequences.

While this case collection was being written, several more cases were added, and by October, 2019, I will have treated well over 150 patients with chronic active toxoplasmosis or advised on their treatment. *In Germany, a cautious estimate of 1% of the population could be actively affected, with considerable room for uncertainty upwards.* This doesn't allow definitive conclusions to the world–wide risk for chronic active toxoplasmosis, but it is obviously not good news.

Symptoms of exhaustion, unclear muscle pains, poor concentration, poor performance and shortness of breath, sweating, depressive moods, aggressive behavioural changes and anxiety are the results, as are accumulated infections resulting from a weakened immune system. In addition to the serious personal illnesses and suffering, high social and economic burdens arise due to chronic toxoplasmosis diseases as a result of numerous diagnostic measures, hospital stays and indirect costs such as long work incapacities or forced retirement.

The severe impairment of the psyche, which already occurs with a positive Toxoplasma detection is associated with an increased risk for a disturbed concentration, a higher accident risk, a higher aggression readiness and even neurological diseases, This not only burdens the individual considerably, but also a whole society in view of the high number of people infected with Toxoplasma gondii.

There is a symptom overlap of chronic active toxoplasmosis with Chronic Fatigue Syndrome (CFS), and this is probably at least a major part of CFS in some patients. These patients could benefit greatly from toxoplasmosis treatment. The earlier assumption that bradyzoites are inactive and harmless has been refuted several times by basic research, but no consequences have yet been drawn and medicine does not yet take into account the fact that we are so far blind to this part of the disease. The current standard tests only detect antibodies to some form of Toxoplasma, the tachyzoites, and often do not indicate active toxoplasmosis requiring treatment.

The tests are not 100% reliable even in an initial infection and there is strong evidence that they become very unreliable in later stages of the disease. This is because the Toxoplasma appear in a different form, bradyzoites, in a chronic progression, which differ strongly from the tachyzoites in their surface structure and which hide in cysts. Therefore, they are not detected by laboratory tests, and in some cases the laboratory values are even completely negative, even though active toxoplasmosis requiring treatment is present.

New, more sensitive test methods, which show a bradyzoite activity and thus also detect a toxoplasmosis in a chronically active form are under development. However, people who now have chronic active toxoplasmosis are often too ill to wait years before these tests become widely available. After exclusion of other causes of disease, a screening by means of questionnaires, as presented here, is a way to uncover these disease processes.

If there is a reasonable suspicion of active toxoplasmosis and other causes of disease have been excluded, antibiotic treatment for 7-10 days is likely to identify cases in which a multiple combination over several weeks is meaningful and promising. Again, this method is not 100% reliable, but it has a high probability of helping sufferers. On the other hand, the strict adherence to still unreliable laboratory values lead doctors to not even consider such a treatment despite severe symptoms. There is no need for specialized departments to treat toxoplasmosis effectively, because every doctor can familiarize himself or herself with this disease.

The known combination therapies are highly effective, but sometimes have to be adjusted or rearranged in the course of treatment due to a decreasing effect or side-effects. Therefore, a close monitoring of patients by the attending physician is crucial. The very high symptom improvements of up to 100%, even after the sometimes very long course of the disease, as well as the quality of life documented in the case studies clearly show what a value toxoplasmosis therapy can be in medical practice.

The parasites cannot be killed by the therapies available so far, but only be weakened to a point that our immune system can regain control. The surviving Toxoplasma can cause relapses after months or years, but such relapses are usually well treatable.

In my opinion, the risks of toxoplasmosis must be assessed much higher than now. Necessary consequences would be to remove Toxoplasma gondii as much as possible from the food cycle and to eat risky foods only after prior freezing, cooking thoroughly or in the case of vegetables, only after they are thoroughly washed.

All health insurance companies should be obliged to offer a toxo-plasmosis screening during pregnancy. In Germany, atypical high-risk Toxoplasma strains have been detected and there is an urgent need for action. Patients must be treated and, in the long term, a much lower level of infection, such as in Northern Europe must be the aim. This would significantly reduce the risk of disease and thus the burden on patients and the healthcare systems.

Good medicine does not begin with technology, but above all with listening and trust, and that makes this profession so unparalleled. A good education, a thorough medical history and physical examination, interest in others, empathy, care and commitment to patients are further indispensable components of the medical work, and it is an extremely fulfilling, beautiful work. Trust is not a one-way street, and as a doctor you have to trust your patients. In my experience, the patients' information on their illnesses is for the most part very detailed, open and honest.

They deserve trust, and collaboration between doctor and patient is not only nicer, but also more effective than a medicine that is exercised "top-down". Technical measures have become an indispensable part of medicine and have greatly improved it, but they are not perfect.

One should not make technical results the sole standard, otherwise there is a great risk that patients whose symptoms cannot be explained technically will automatically be declared "psychosomatic cases". Psychosomatic diagnoses are then too often pronounced or degenerate to an excuse, and that just should not happen. It can be timeconsuming and laborious to work out the right diagnoses, but at the end of the work often comes a patient whose condition is significantly alleviated or cured - and a relieved doctor.

Without the excellent effects of toxoplasmosis therapies, I would have stopped treatments early, and there would have been no checklist, no case collection, no book on the subject either, but only many patients whom I could not have helped. These therapies *are* effective and have become an indispensable part of my work, and I wanted to tell you about them.

I hope to reach as many affected people and their doctors as possible, and maybe university medicine will devote more attention to this topic as well. It would benefit many people.

Dr. med. U. Auf der Straße, 04.11.2019

19. Technical terms

Bradyzoites (brady Greek for "slow") They represent the survival form of Toxoplasma in the host organism. They have a built-in biological camouflage function in that their surface structure is almost completely changed compared to the tachyzoites, so that antibodies against tachyzoites cannot affect them. Bradyzoites create permanent cysts in the host cells, which largely consist of the "interior outfit" of these cells. There they are very difficult for the immune system to find and can continue to multiply. Bradyzoites themselves cause almost no antibody production.

Their metabolism is slowed down and it has only been known for a few years that they, too, can divide. Bradyzoites do not rest, as previously assumed, but represent an active, serious burden to the host. When the host's immune system is temporarily weakened, they can transform into tachyzoites, increase their rate of reproduction, and continue to spread in the organism. Improperly cooked meat containing bradyzoite cysts is infectious.

CD8 cells These specialized white blood cells are indispensable for combating pathogens found *in* our cells. They are important opponents of Toxoplasma. They are able to simultaneously produce 4 different messenger substances for the immune system (interferons). However, they can become exhausted if exposure to Toxoplasma is too high or if other diseases such as EBV or CMV are coped with at the same time. (see pp. 59-60). They then lose the ability to form two of these interferons. This weakens the immune system and allows for increased conversion of bradyzoites into tachyzoites. The toxoplasmosis can then change to a more active state.

Oocysts: They are excreted in the faeces of infected cats and are protective covers containing the eggs of the Toxoplasma, the sporozoites. Oocysts are very stable, can last for several years in the ground and survive most disinfectants. They are present in large quantities in our environment (see page 47)

Sporozoites: the eggs of Toxoplasma. They mature in the oocysts and become infectious about two days after the oocysts are shed.

Tachyzoites (tachy is Greek for "fast"): this is the attack form of Toxoplasma. They are highly mobile, can rapidly penetrate cells of the host and reach almost all tissues. They multiply in the host cells at high speed in pseudo-cysts until the host cell bursts (blasts) under a load of several hundred tachyzoites. They can control our immune system, even survive in macrophages (phagocytes) and use them to get into the particularly secure central nervous system of the host. When tachyzoites are under too much pressure from the immune system, they convert to bradyzoites and survive in tissue cysts throughout their lives. If the immune system of the host is weakened, they can transform back to tachyzoits any time.

20. References

1) Aguirre-Cruz L., Calderon M., and Sotelo J.: *Colchicine Decreases the Infection by Toxoplasma gondii in Cultured Glia Cells*. The Journal of Parasitology Vol. 82, No. 2 (Apr., 1996), pp. 325-327

2)   Alavi S.M., Alavi L. : *Treatment of toxoplasmic lymphadenitis with cotrimoxazole: double-blind, randomized clinical trial.*   Int J Infect Dis. 2010 Sep;14 Suppl 3:e67-9. doi: 10.1016/j.ijid.2009.11.015. Epub 2010 Mar 2.

3)   Aliberti, J., D. Jankovic, and A. Sher. 2004.   *Turning it on and off: regulation of dendritic cell function in Toxoplasma gondii infection.* Immunol. Rev.201:26–34.

4) Aramini J.J., Stephen C., Dubai J.P., Engelstoft C., Schwantje H., Ribble C.S. *Potential contamination of drinking water with Toxoplasma gondii oocysts.* Epidemic Infect. 1999 April; 122(2):305-15

5) Assimakopoulos, S.F., Stamouli V., Dimitropoulou D., Spiliopoulou A., Panos G., Anastassiou M., Marangos M., Spiliopoulou I.: *Toxoplasma gondii meningoencephalitis without cerebral MRI findings in a patient with ulcerative colitis under immunsuppressive treatment.* Infection 5/2015

6) Bhadra Rajarshi,   Khan Imtiaz A. 2012:   *Redefining Chronic Toxoplasmosis - A T Cell Exhaustion Perspective.* Department of Microbiology, Immunology and Tropical Medicine, George Washington University, Washington, D.C., United States of America PLoS Pathogens, 8(10), article number 1002903.

7) Behan W.M.H., Behan P., P.O., Draper I.T. & Williams H., (1983). *Does Toxoplasma gondii cause polymyositis?* Acta neuropathologica, 61, 246-52

8) Berverly J.K.A, Beattie, C.P. (1958) *Glandular toxoplasmosis. A survey of 30 cases.* Lancet, ii, 379-84

9) Blais J., Tardif C., and Chamberlain S.: *Effect of clindamycin on intracellular replication, protein synthesis, and infectivity of Toxoplasma gondii.* Antimicrob Agents Chemother. 1993 Dec; 37(12): 2571–2577.

10) Bretagne S.: *Molecular diagnostics in clinical parasitology and mycology: limits of the current polymerase chain reaction (PCR) assays and interest of the real-time PCR assays.* Clin Microbiol Infect 2003, 9:505-11.

11) Carme B., Bissuel F., Ajzenberg D., Bouyne R., Aznar C., Demar M., Louvel D., Bourbigot M., Peneau C., Neron P. and Darde M.L: *Severe Acquired Toxoplasmosis in Immunocompetent Adult Patients in French Guiana.* J Clin Microbiol. 2002 Nov; 40(11): 4037–4044.

12) Coccaro E.F., Royce Lee, Maureen W.Groer, Adem Can, Mary Coussons-Read and T.T. Postolache: *Toxoplasma gondii Infection: Relationship With Aggression in Psychiatric subjects.* The Journal of Clinical Psychiatry 2016; 77 (3): 334-341

13) Colinot D.L., Garbuz T., Wang L., Rice S.E., Sullivan W.J. Jr., Arrizabalanga G., JerdeT.J.: *The common parasite Toxoplasma gondii induces prostatic inflammation and microglandular hyperplasia in a mouse model.* Prostrate, 2017 Jul;77(10):1066-1075. doi: 10.1002/pros.23362. Epub 2017 May 12.

14) Cook A.J.C., Gilbert R.E., Buffolano W., Zuffrey J., Petersen E., Jenum P.A., Foulon W., Semprini A.E., Dunn D.T. & *European Research Network on Congenital Toxoplasmosis Sources of Toxoplasma infection in pregnant women: European multicentre case control study* BMJ 2015, Juli; 321, 142-147

15) Courret N, Darche S, Sonigo P, Milon G, Buzoni-Gâtel D, Tardieux I. : *CD11c- and CD11b-expressing mouse leukocytes transport single Toxoplasma gondii tachyzoites to the brain.* Blood 2006 Jan 1; 107(1): 309–316.

16) Cuturic M., Hayat G.R., Vogler C.A., Velasques A. *Toxoplasmic polymyositis revisited: case report and review of literature.* Neuromuscul Disord. 1997 Sep; 7 (6-7): 390-6

17) Dalimi A. and Abdoli A. *Latent Toxoplasmosis and Human.* Iran J Parasitol. 2012; 7(1): 1-17

18) Dannemann B., McCutchan J.A., Israelski D., et al. Treatment of toxoplasmic encephalitis in Patients with AIDS. *A randomized trial comparing pyrimthamine plus Clindamycin to Pyrimethamin plus Sulfa- diazine.* Ann Intern Med 1992, 116: 33-43

19) Denkers, E. Y., and B. A. Butcher. 2005. *Sabotage and exploitation in macrophages parasitized by intracellular protozoans.* Trends Parasitol. 21: 35–41.

20) Desmonts G., Naot Y., Remington J.S. *Immunoglobulin M immuno- sorbent agglutination assay for diagnosis of infectious diseases. Diagnosis of acute congenital and acquired Toxoplasma infections.* J. clin Microbiol. 1981; 14: 544-549

21) Di Cristina, M., Dou, Z., Lunghi, M., Kannan, G., Huynh, M. H., McGovern, O. L., .. Carruthers, V. B. (2017). Toxoplasma depends on lysosomal consumption of autophagosomes for persistent infection. Nature Microbiology,2, [17096]. DOI: 10.1038/ nmicrobiol. 2017.96

22) Dickerson F., Wilcox H.C., Adamos M., Katsafanas E., Khushalani S., Origoni A., Savage C., Schweinfurth L., Stallings C., Sweeney K., Yolken R.: *Suicide attempts and markers of immune response in individuals with serious mental illness.* J Psychiatr Res. 2017 Apr;87:37-43. Doi: 10.1016/j.jpsychires.2016.11.011. Epub 2016 Dec 1.

23) Dogan N., Kabukcuoglu S., Vardareli E. *Toxoplasmic Hepatitis in an Immunocompetent Patient.* Türkiye Parazitoloji Dergisi, 31 (4): 260-263, 2007

24) Dubey J.P., Gamble H.R., Hill D., Sreekumar C., Romand S., Thulliez P.: *High prevalence of viable Toxoplasma Gondii in market weight pigs from a farm in Massachusetts.* J. Parasitol., 88(6), 2002, pp. 1234–1238

25) Eyles D., Coleman N. *Synergistic effect of sulphadiazine and daraprim against experimental toxoplasmosis in the mouse.* Antibiot. Chemother. 1953; 3: 483-90

26) Ferguson D.J., Hutchinson W.M. Petersen E. 1989 *Tissue cyst rupture in mice chronically infected with Toxoplasma gondii. An Immunocytochemical and ultrastructural study.* Parasitol Res 75: 599 – 603

27) Fischer H.G., Nitzen B., Reichmann G., Haddig u. *Cytokin responses induced by Toxoplasma gondii in atrocytes and microglial cells* Eur J Immunol 1997 Jun;27(6):1539-48.

28) Flegr, J. (2007). *Effects of Toxoplasma on human behavior.* Schizophr. Bull. 33, 757–760.

29) Flegr J.: *Influence of latent Toxoplasma infection on human personality, physiology and morphology: pros and cons of the Toxoplasma-human model in studying the manipulation hypothesis.* J. Exp. Biol. 2013; 216 (Pt 1): 127 -33

30) Flegr J, Escudero DQ. *Impaired health status and increased incidence of diseases in Toxoplasma-seropositive subjects - an explorative cross-sectional study. Parasitology* 2016; 143: 1974-1989.

31) Jaroslav Flegr, Joseph Prandota, Michaela Sovicˇkova´, Zafar H. Israili: *Toxoplasmosis – A Global Threat. Correlation of Latent Toxoplasmosis with Specific Disease Burden in a Set of 88 Countries.* PloS One 2014 Mar 24;9(3):e90203. doi: 10.1371/journal.pone.0090203. eCollection 2014.

32) Frenkel J.K.: *Adoptive Immunity to Intracellular Infection*
J Immunol June 1, 1967, 98 (6) 1309-1319

33) Frenkel J.K., Smith D.D.: *Immunization of cats against shedding of Toxoplasma oocysts.* J. Parasitol. 1982 Oct;68(5):744-8.

34) Ganji M., Tan A., Maitar, Michael, Weldon-Linne, M., Weisenberg E., and Douglas P.R.(*2003*) *Gastric Toxoplasmosis in a Patient With Acquired Immunodeficiency Syndrome A Case Report and Review of the Literature.* Archives of Pathology & Laboratory Medicine: June 2003, Vol. 127, No. 6, pp. 732-734.

35) Gigley, J.P., Bhadra R., Khan I.A. *CD8 T Cells and Toxoplasma gondii: A New Paradigm* Journal of Parasitology Research Volume 2011 (2011) Article ID 243796, 9 pages

36) Gras L., Gilbert R.E., Wallon M., Peyron F., Cortina-Borja M.: *Duration of the IgM response in women acquiring Toxoplasma gondii during pregnancy: implications for clinical practice and cross-sectional incidence studies.* Epidemie Infect. 2004 Jun; 132(3): 541-548

37) Greenlee J.E., Johnson W.D., Jr, Campa, J.F., Adelman L.S., Sande M.A.: *Adult toxoplasmosis presenting as polymyositis and cerebellar ataxia.* Ann Intern Med. 1975; 82: 367-371

38) Grigg et al., 2001: *Experimentally induced sexual recombination in the cat* Science 294, 161-5

39) Havlicek J., Gasova Z.G., Smith A.P., Zvara K., Flegr J. *Decrease of psychomotor performance in subjects with latent "asymptomatic" toxoplasmosis.* Parasitology 2001 May; 122(Pt 5): 515-20

40) Hökelek M. MD, PhD; 2015 Chief Editor: Michael Stuart Bronze, MD: *Toxoplasmosis Medication* In: Medscape Drugs & Diseases

41) Helieh S. Oz, DVM, PhD, AGAF: *Toxoplasma gondii (Toxoplasmosis)* Authors, Second Edition: Montoya, J.G, Couvreur J., Leport, C. In: antimicrobiobe.org

42) Hermes G., Ajioka J., Kelly K., Mui E., Roberts F., Kasza K., Mayr T., Kirisits M., Wollmann R., Ferguson D., Roberts C., Hwang J., Trendler T., Kennan R., Suzuki Y., Reardon C., Hickey W., Chen L., McLeod R.: *Neurological and behavioral abnormalities, ventricular dilatation, altered cellular functions, inflammation, and neuronal injury in brains of mice due to common, persistent, parasitic infection.* Journal of Neuroinflammation. 2008, 5:48 doi:10.1186/1742-2094-5-48

43) Herrmann D.C., Pantchev N., Globokar Vrhovec M., Barutzki D., Wilking H., Fröhlich A., Lüder C.G.K., F.J. Conraths F.J., Schares G.: *Atypical Toxoplasma gondii genotypes identified in oocysts shed by cats in Germany.* International Journal for Parasitology 40 (2010) 285–292

44) Hill D., Dubey J.P.: *Toxopasma gondii: transmission, diagnosis and prevention* Clin Microbiol Infect. 2002; 8: 634-640

45) Ho-Yen D.O. : *Toxoplasmosis in humans.* J Roy Soc Med 1990; 83: 571-2

46) Ho-Yen D.O., Joss A.W.L., Balfour A.H., Smyth E.T.M., Baird D., Chatterton J.M.W.: *Use of the polymerase chain reaction to detect Toxoplasma gondii in human blood samples.* J Clin Pathol 1992; 45: 910-913

47) Janků, J., 1923. *Pathogenesis and pathologic anatomy of the "congenital coloboma" of the macula lutea in an eye of normal size, with microscopic detection of parasites in the retina.* Cas Lek Ses. 1923, 62: 1021-1027.

48) Jacobs L.: *The occurrence of Toxoplasma infection in the absence of demonstrable antibodies* In book: Proceedings of the first international Congress of Parasitology

49) Jean M., Chatterton W., McDonagh S., Spence Neil and Ho-Yen Darrel-O. *Changes in Toxoplasma diagnosis* Journal of Medical Microbiology 2011, 60 (Pt 12): 1762-1766

50) Johnson Alan P. *Methicillin-resistant Staphylococcus aureus: the European landscape* J.Antimicrobial Chemotherapy, Volume 66, Issue suppl 4, 1 May 2011, Pages iv43–iv48

51) Kabelitz, H.J.: *Abdominelle Symptome bei postnatal erworbener Toxoplasmose.* Deutsche medizinische Wochenschrift 1959 Vol.84 No.31 pp.1379-84, 1404 ref.17

52) Kotula A.W., Dubey J.P., Sharar A.K., Andrews C.D., Shen S.K., Lindsay D.S.: *Effect of Freezing on Infectivity of Toxoplasma gondii* Tissue Cysts in Pork. J Food Prot. 1991;54:687-90.

53) Kuruca L , Klun I., Uzelac A., Nicolic A., Bobic B., Simin S., Lalosevic V., Lalosevic D., Djurkovic-Djakovic O.: *Detection of Toxoplasma gondii in naturally infected domestic pigs in Northern Serbia.* Parasitol Res. 2017 Nov;116(11):3117-3123. doi: 10.1007/s00436-017-5623-7. Epub 2017 Sep 27.

54) Leal, F.E., Cavazanna, C.S., de Andrale,H.F.Jr., Galisteo, A.J.Jr, de Mendonca, J.S., Kallas, E.G.,*Toxoplasma gondii Pneumonia in Immunocompetent Subjects: Case Report and Review* Clinical Infectious Diseases, Volume 44, Issue 6, 15 March 2007, Pages e62–e66

55) Luft, B.J. & Remington J.S. (1985). *Toxoplasmosis of the central nervous system.* Current Clinical Topics in Infectious Diseases, ed J.S. Remington, M.n. Swartz, pp. 315-58. New York: McGraw-Hill

56) Mavin S., Ashburn D., Chatterton J.M.W., Evans R., Joss A.W.L. and Ho-Yen D.O. (2000)*Patterns of Toxoplasma infection during 1996-1999.* Scieh Wkly Rep 34, 278-280

57) Montazeri M., Mehrzadi S., Sharif M., Sarvi S., Shahdin S., Daryani A.: *Activities of anti-Toxoplasma drugs and compounds against tissue cysts in the last three decades (1987 to 2017), a systematic review. Parasitol research* 2018 Oct;117(10):3045-3057. doi: 10.1007/s00436-018-6027-z. Epub 2018 Aug 8.

58) Montoya J.G., Jordan R. Lingamneni S. Berry G.J., Remington J.S. : *Toxoplasmic myokarditis and polymyositis in patients with acquired toxoplasmosis diagnosed during life* Clin Infect Dis. 1997; 24 676-683

59) Montoya J.M, Liesenfeld O. : *Toxoplasmosis.* Lancet. 2004; 363: 1965-1976

60) Naviaux, Robert K. Naviaux, Jane C., Li, Kefeng, Bright, A. Taylor, Alaynick, William A. , Wang, Lin, Baxter, Asha, Nathan, Neil, Anderson. Wayne and Gordon, Eric: *Metabolic features of chronic fatigue syndrome* PNAS 2016 September, 113 (37) E5472-E5480.

61) Nicolle C, Manceaux L. : Sur un protozoaire nouveau du gondi. C R Seances Acad Sci. 1909;148:369–372.

62) Nilamadhab Kar, Baikunthanath Misra: *Toxoplasma seropositivity and depression: case report* BMC Psychiatry 2004 4:1

63) Paspalaki P., E. Mihailidou, M. Bitsori, D. Tsagkaraki, E. Mantzouranis: *Polymyositis and myocarditis associated with acquired toxoplasmosis in an immunocompetent girl.* Department of Pediatrics, University General Hospital, University of Crete, School of Health Science. BMC Musculoskelet Disord. 2001; 2: 8. Published online 2001 Nov 20.

64) Pappas G., Roussos N. & Falagas M.E. (2009) : *Toxoplasmosis snapshots: global status of Toxoplasma gondii seroprevalence and implications for pregnantcy and congenital toxoplasmosis* Int J Parasitol 39, 1385-1394

65) Pernas L, Adomako-Ankomah Y, Shastri AJ, Ewald SE, Treeck M, Boyle JP, Boothroyd JC: *Toxoplasma effector MAF1 mediates recruitment ho mitochondria and impacts the host response.* PLoS Biol. 2014 Apr; 12(4):e1001845.

66) Prusa A.R., Hayde M., Pollak A., Herkner K.R.,Kasper D.C.: *Evaluation of the Liaison Automated Testing System for Diagnosis of Congenital Toxoplasmosis.* Clin Vaccine Immunol. 2012 Nov; 19(11): 1859-1863

67) Prusa A.R., Kasper D.C., Pollak A., Gleiss A., Waldhoer T., Hayde M.: *The Austrian Toxoplasmosis Register, 1992-2008* in: *Clinical Infectious Diseases,* Volume 60, Issue 2, 15 January 2015, Pages e4–e10,

68) Remington J.S., Mc Leod R., Thulliez P. et al.: *Toxoplasmosis.* In: Infectious Diseases of the Fetus an Newborn infant, WB Saunders; 2001 pp 205 – 346 Editors Remington J.S., Klein J.

69) Remington J.S, Miller M.J., Brownlee I.E. *IgM antibodies in acute Toxoplasmosis.* II Prevalence and significance in aquired cases. J. Lab Clin Med. 1968; 71 855-866 (PubMed)

70) Remington J.S.: *Toxoplasmosis in the adult.* Bull N Y Acad Med. 1974; 50: 211-227

71) Sabin A.B., Feldman H.A.1948. *Dyes as microchemical indicators of a new immunity phenomenon affecting a protozoon parasite (Toxoplasma).* Science 108: 660-663.

72) Schares G., Herrmann, D.C., Pantchev N., Globokar Vrhovec M., Barutzki D., Wilking H., Fröhlich A., Leder C.G.K., und Conrads F.J. : *Erster Nachweis atypischer Toxoplasma gondii - Genotypen in Deutschland* In: ToxoNet 01, www.zoonose.net

73) Schölkopf, M.: Das Gesundheitswesen im internationalen Vergleich. Gesundheitssystemvergleich und die europäische Gesundheitspolitik

74) Seon-Kyeong Kim and John C. Boothroyd: *Stage-Specific Expression of Surface Antigens by Toxoplasma gondii as a Mechanism to Facilitate Parasite Persistence* J. Clin Immunol 2005; 174:8038-8048

75) Sharpe, M.C., Archard L., Banatvala J., Borysiewicz l.K., Clare A.W., David A., Edwards R., Hawton K.E.H et al (1991): *Chronic fatigue Syndrom: Guidelines for research* Journal of the Royal Society Medicine, 84, 115-21

76) Sinai, A. P., and K. A. Joiner. 1997. *Safe haven: the cell biology of nonfusogenic pathogen vacuoles.* Annu. Rev. Microbiol. 51: 415–462.

77) Smith J.E., Mc Neil G., Zhang Y.W., Dutton G., Biswas-Hughes G., Applefordt P.: *Serological Recognition of Toxoplasma gondii Cyst Antigens.* Curr Top Microbiol Immunol. 1996;219:67-73.

78) Suzuki Y. and Remington J.S. : *Dual regulation of resistance against Toxoplasma gondii infection by Lyt-2+ and Lyt-1+, L3T4+ T cells in mice.* Journal of Immunology, vol. 140, no. 11, pp. 3943–3946, 1988.

79) Suzuki Y., Orellana M.A., Schreiber R.D., Remington J.S. : *Interferon-gamma: the major mediator of resistance against Toxoplasma gondii.* Science. 1988 Apr 22;240(4851):516-8.

80) *Syn Genevieve, Anderson Denise and Blackwell Jenefer M.:* Toxoplasma gondii *Infection Is Associated with Mitochondrial Dysfunction* in Vitro. Front Cell Infect Microbiol. 2017;7:512 Published online 2017 Dec 12.

81) Torrey E.F., Bartok J.J., Yolken R.H.: *Toxoplasma gondii and other risk factors for schizophrenia: an update.* Schizophren Bull. 2012; 38(3): 642-647

82) Torrey E.F., Yolken R.H.: *Toxoplasma oocysts as a public health problem. Trends in Parasitology 2013 Aug;29(8):380-4. 2013 Jul 9.*

83) Townsend J.J., Wolinsky J.S., Baringer J.R., Johnson P.C.: *Acquired toxoplasmosis. A neglected cause of treatable nervous system disease.* Arch Neurol. 1975 May;32(5):335–343.

84) Watts E., Zhao Y., Dhara A., Eller B., Patwardhan A.R. and Anthony P.S.: *Novel Approach Reveal that Toxoplasma gondii Bradyzoites within Tissue Cysts Are Dynamic and Replicating Entities in Vivo* (2015). Microbiology, Immunology and Molecular Genetics Faculty Publications. Paper 67

85) Weiss, Louis M. and Dubey, Jitender P.: *Toxoplasmosis: A history of clinical observation* Int J parasitol 2009 Jul 1: 39(8): 895-901

86) Weiss, LM, Perlman DC, Sherman J, Tanowitz H, Wittner M. *Isospora belli infection: treatment with pyrimethamine.* Ann Intern Med. Sep 15, 1988; 109(6):474-475. Available at pubmed/3261956. www.ncbi.nlm.nih.gov

87) White PD. *What Causes Prolonged Fatigue after Infectious Mononucleosis: And Does It Tell Us Anything about Chronic Fatigue Syndrome?* J. Infect Dis 2007;196:4–5

88) Wilking H., Thamm M., Stark K., Aebischer T. and Seeber F.: *Prevalence, incidence estimations, and risk factors of Toxoplasma gondii infection in Germany: a representative, cross-sectional, serological study* In: Nature.com / Scientific Reports 6, Article number: 22551 (2016)

89) Wolf A, Cowen D. Granulomatous encephalomyelitis due to a protozoan (*Toxoplasma* or *Encephalitozoon*). II identification of a case from the literature. Bull Neur Inst NY. 1938;7:266–290.

90) Wolf A, Cowen D, Paige B. Human toxoplasmosis: occurrence in infants as an encephalomyelitis verification by transmission to animals. Science. 1939A;89:226–227.

91) Yagmur F., Yasar S., Ozcan Temel H., Cavusoglu M.: *May Toxoplasma gondii increase suicide attempt ? - preliminary results in Turkish subjects* Forens Sci Int. 2010; 199: 15-17

92) Yolken R.H., Bachmann S., Ruslanova I., Lillehoj E., Ford G., Torrey E.F., Schroeder J.: *Antibodies to Toxoplasma gondii in individuals with first-episode schizophrenia.* Clin Infect Dis 2001 Mar 1; 32(5):842

93) Xiao J., Prandovszky E., Kannan G., Pletnikov M.V., Dickerson F., Severance E.G., Yolken R.H. : *Toxoplasma gondii: Biological Parameters of the Connection to Schizophrenia.* Schizophr Bull. 2018 Aug 20;44(5):983-992. doi: 10.1093/schbul/sby082.

94) Yolken R.H., Torrey E.F. *Are some cases of psychosis caused by microbial agents ? A review of the evidence.* Mol Psychiatry. 2008; 13: 470-479

95) Zhang Y.W., Fraser A., Balfour A.H., Wreghitt T.G., Gray J.J., Smith J.E. : *Serological reactivity against cyst and tachyzoite antigens of Toxoplasma gondii determined by Fast - Elisa* J. J. clin Pathol 1995;48:908-91